Tapping the Healer Within

Using Thought Field Therapy to instantly conquer your fears, anxieties and emotional distress

ROGER CALLAHAN
with Richard Trubo

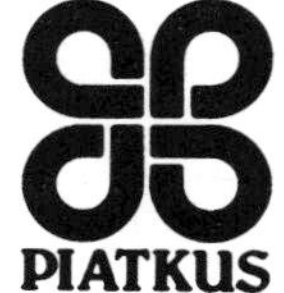

PIATKUS

First published in Great Britain in 2001 by Piatkus Books
Reprinted 2002, 2003, 2004, 2005 (twice), 2006, 2007, 2008 (twice)

A CIP catalogue record for this book
is available from the British Library

ISBN 978-0-7499-2232-0

Printed and bound in Great Britain by
CPI Mackays, Chatham, ME5 8TD

Papers used by Piatkus Books are natural, renewable and recyclable products made from wood grown in sustainable forests and certified in accordance with the rules of the Forest Stewardship Council.

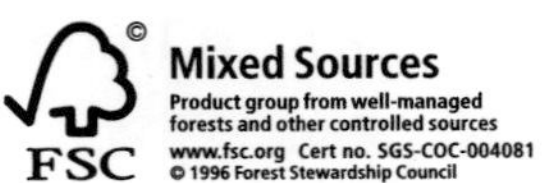

Piatkus Books
An imprint of
Little, Brown Book Group
100 Victoria Embankment
London EC4Y 0DY

An Hachette Livre UK Company
www.hachettelivre.co.uk

www.piatkus.co.uk

This book is dedicated to my wife,
Joanne Somavia De Laveaga Callahan.

—Roger J. Callahan

CONTENTS

FOREWORD

In *Tapping the Healer Within*, Dr. Roger Callahan explains his groundbreaking health technique of Thought Field Therapy in an easy-to-follow, step-by-step process. He shows how to overcome a variety of common problems, such as phobias, compulsions, trauma, anxiety, addictive urges, depression, obsessions, jet lag, and physical pain.

He clearly explains how anyone can learn his technique quickly and apply it instantly. The illustrations demonstrate exactly how and where to apply his method. He describes the breathing techniques and treating points so well that you can easily understand how to treat yourself.

Even such hard to overcome difficulties as claustrophobia and fear of spiders and of flying are discussed, and the specific treatment for each of these conditions is shown. Dr. Callahan explains how anger and rage cause physical problems and suggests how to cope with them. Even if you have a complex case, this method works. A psychotherapist for over fifty years, Dr. Callahan has been using and updating his Thought Field Therapy technique for the last twenty years. It is now being used and proven effective by his students and colleagues worldwide.

This book is an invaluable tool for helping anyone suffering from a psychological or physical problem get back onto the road of optimal health.

—Dr. Earl Mindell

ACKNOWLEDGMENTS

EACH TIME I am called upon to write an acknowledgment for my work, I am immediately moved to thank the unknown genius of the Orient who, over five thousand years ago, first discovered the meridian (acupuncture) system.

The other person whose discoveries play a role in my work is a brilliant chiropractor from Detroit, George Goodheart, D.C. Dr. Goodheart discovered and developed the field of applied kinesiology (AK). It was some of his basic findings that allowed me, with the help of the meridian system, to develop my causal diagnostic system, which then made it possible for me to discover the highly successful treatments, or algorithms, for the numerous problems whose solutions are presented in this book.

I also thank Robert Blaich, D.C., and David Walther, D.C., for their superb teaching of the hundred-hour course in AK that I was privileged to attend. Dr. Blaich also did early work in establishing the value and power of my concept of psychological reversal.

It is important to state that the two links—acupuncture and applied kinesiology—in my discovery are not at all responsible for my new findings; they are solely my own, as are any unwitting mistakes.

My discoveries are now receiving strong scientific support through the use of a technology everyone will be hearing more about in the near future. It is called Heart Rate Variability (HRV). One of the important contributions of HRV, besides being a powerful and objective test of therapy effectiveness, is that it is the best predictor of mortality for all conditions. I want to thank Fuller Royal, M.D., of Las Vegas for finding that my discoveries make a powerful impact on this measurement. I also want to thank Peter Julian, Sallie Baugh, and Rick Roncka for helping us to understand some of the technical aspects of HRV. As far as I can determine, mine is the only therapy that dramatically improves HRV—and these changes are typically accomplished in minutes. The HRV results suggest my discoveries may extend and protect the lives of those suffering from heart or other life-threatening conditions. We eagerly look forward to additional research on this important matter.

I want to thank my wife, Joanne Somavia De Laveaga Callahan, for her unending support and love—I couldn't do it without her. To our top level trainees in Thought Field Therapy, I give a salute for all their help and support: Yoshinori Takasaki, M.D.; Jill Strunk, Ed.D.; Norma Schenck, LCSW; Stephen Daniel, Ph.D.; Gale Joslin, Ph.D.; Liz Joslin, LCSW; Monica Pignotti, CSW; Caroline Sakai, Ph.D.; Jenny Edwards, Ph.D.; Luis Jorge Gonzalez, Ph.D.; Mark Steinberg, Ph.D.; Frank Patton, Ph.D.; Rose Patton, R.N.; Rick Moses, Ph.D.; Alex Loyd, Ph.D.; Joel Wade, Ph.D.; and Mary Cowley, Ph.D.

Richard and I gratefully thank our dynamic New York agent, Jane Dystel. Jane performed acts of unusual skill and heroism in getting this book the recognition it deserves.

My deep thanks to a very special and gifted writer, Richard Trubo. Much gratitude is due to our very talented editor, Judith McCarthy, who made this enterprise a most enjoyable one. Richard and I also thank Judith for her basic and helpful suggestions and excellent contributions to this book.

—*Roger J. Callahan*

part one

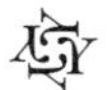

ALL ABOUT THOUGHT FIELD THERAPY

1

THOUGHT FIELD THERAPY: A REVOLUTIONARY WAY OF HEALING

IMAGINE BEING IN emotional distress, but finding rapid relief in just minutes. Picture yourself overwhelmed by chronic stress, addicted to nicotine, or crippled by a fear of flying—but eradicating these or other kinds of debilitating problems almost instantaneously.

The answer to the negative emotions in your life is a powerful treatment called Thought Field Therapy (TFT). It represents a revolutionary advance in the way psychological disturbances are perceived and managed. Tens of thousands of people worldwide have already used TFT to conquer their fears, eliminate their compulsions, recover from broken relationships, put an end to procrastination, and quiet their anger and grief. It has provided them with emotional renewal, rapidly and safely, without long-term psychotherapy and without medications. There are no risks. There are no side effects.

This program can work for you, too.

WHAT IS TFT?

Thought Field Therapy is different from any other psychological treatment that you've ever used. The therapeutic process itself is completely unique. So is the scientific foundation on which it's based. And so are the unprecedented results it can produce.

TFT is a system that accesses and resolves the essence and the root cause of your problem, whether it is a phobia, anger, a bad habit, trauma, anxiety, guilt, or grief. These negative emotions are condensed information in energy form, bound in what I call a *Thought Field* (we'll explain the concept of the Thought Field more thoroughly later). The *active information* in this Thought Field creates distress in your life by disrupting the body's internal energy flow, causing psychological upheaval that sabotages your emotional well-being.

A key to the treatment is influencing the body's bioenergy field by tapping with your fingers on specific points on the body located along energy meridians. In a user-friendly process that you'll learn in detail, you'll think about the particular psychological concern that is troubling you and then quantify the intensity of the emotional upset you're feeling (on a scale from 1 to 10). Next, you will tap on specific points on the body in a particular sequence. As that happens, you will eliminate imbalances in the body's energy system, and in the process, weaken and even eradicate negative emotions and the symptoms of psychological distress. Thanks to new research using technology that can monitor the body's autonomic nervous system, we can now scientifically measure and quantify the systemic changes that TFT produces. Clearly, TFT heals at the most fundamental level—and it happens almost instantaneously.

Over the years, I've created and fine-tuned this definition of TFT:

TFT is a treatment for psychological disturbances which provides a code that, when applied to a psychological problem the individual is attuned to, will eliminate perturbations in the Thought Field, the fundamental cause of all negative emotions. This code is elicited through TFT's causal diagnostic procedure, through which the TFT algorithms were developed.

Of course, there are some components of this definition that you may not understand yet. But by the time you've finished reading this book, it will make sense to you. More important, you'll experience its power in resolving whatever psychological (and even physiological) difficulties you may be experiencing. It can work for you in minutes, as it already has for many thousands of people. In short, it can turn your life around.

A LITTLE BACKGROUND

As I'm sure you've already realized, Thought Field Therapy represents a radical shift in the way psychological distress is treated. For most of this century, talk therapy has been the traditional and accepted path to emotional healing. In fact, until about two decades ago, I was practicing this kind of mainstream psychotherapy. I was also teaching it at the college level. At the same time, however, I was deeply troubled by its shortcomings.

My own background couldn't have been more conventional. After earning a Ph.D. in clinical psychology at Syracuse University, I was Associate Professor and Director of Psychological Services and Research at Eastern Michigan University, and then I taught courses at the University of Michigan before entering private practice. I served as President of the American Academy of Psychologists in Marital and Family Therapy. Back then, my résumé clearly had a traditional bent.

Nevertheless, I've always sought out new approaches to healing. I was a pioneer in cognitive therapy and clinical hypnotherapy, which I hoped could help rescue patients from the failings that I had seen with conventional psychotherapy. Like many psychotherapists, I wanted my clients to get better. I wanted to deliver them from the distress in their lives and help them function normally again. But I felt strongly that, as a profession, modern psychotherapy was letting patients down. Whether we were treating them for depression, phobias, or a shattered relationship, too many clients seem entrapped in years of expensive psychotherapy, talking endlessly about their life circumstances. They'd painfully relive their trauma. They'd often blame something or someone in their past for their current troubles. But at the end of the day—or the year—they had nothing to show for it. They simply weren't being helped. Not only did they continue to spin their wheels, but they also became stuck even deeper in an emotional quagmire. I sometimes felt that my fellow therapists and I were teaching patients only that they could take a hell of a lot more misery than they had thought they could!

I certainly wasn't alone in embracing this bleak perspective of my profession. Some of my fellow psychologists and I often discussed our dismal track records. We agreed that only a small percentage of our patients ever got better. They felt the same frustration I did. They conceded that traditional approaches simply didn't work for most people, and that their own disappointment was exceeded only by the disillusionment and sometimes resentment of their patients. But at the same time, here's what most of them told me: "We're providing our patients with their best chance for healing, whatever the shortcomings of the treatment may be. A small number of success stories is better than none at all." Maybe so. But I was still discouraged, and so were my patients who weren't getting well.

Unlike most of my colleagues, however, I continued to look for something new. I believed there had to be a better way. So I explored innovative therapeutic approaches outside of mainstream psychotherapy. I became passionate about finding a different and more effective therapeutic approach. Through that journey, TFT was born.

MARY'S STORY

Thought Field Therapy grew directly out of my frustration in treating Mary, a patient in her late thirties. Mary was the mother of two, and she had struggled with a severe water phobia since infancy. In fact, she had the most intense fear of water I had seen in my thirty years of practice at that point. It had left her almost paralyzed, incapable of even the most mundane activities. She couldn't take baths in a full tub. She couldn't even bathe her children. Yes, she did take showers, but they were very brief and extremely stressful. Every time it rained, she became absolutely terrified, refusing to set foot outside of her home. She lived in California, but even on the sunniest, most picturesque days, she couldn't drive on Pacific Coast Highway because just the sight of the ocean terrified her. (I remember Mary telling me that she was grateful for the movie *Jaws*, because after seeing that film, her children stopped begging her to take them to the beach!) At night, she had horrifying nightmares that she was being dropped into the ocean by an indefinable, mysterious force, or that water was "getting her."

By 1980, I had been working with Mary for more than a year, using every conventional psychotherapeutic technique I knew. Each approach, however, failed miserably. Mary and I tried rational-emotive therapy, client-centered therapy, cognitive therapy, behavior therapy, hypnosis, relaxation training, biofeedback, systematic desensitization . . . nothing worked. Absolutely nothing.

Like all my colleagues who treated phobias, I forced Mary to confront her fears head-on. Sure, this method can produce anxiety so intense that, in some patients, it can cause post-traumatic stress disorder. Some people feel shell-shocked, as though they have been through a war. But, like Mary, they rarely get better. They are almost never cured. In fact, at that time I had never seen a person whose phobias were completely eradicated. At least some trace of distress always lingered. As frustrated as I felt, my phobic patients were devastated.

Actually, Mary did show signs of a little improvement. After a few months, she had progressed to the point where she could sit anxiously at the edge of the pool outside my home office and dangle her feet in the shallow end. It took real courage for her to even get to that point. However, she felt absolutely terrible each time she would inch her way to the side of the pool. Once there, she could never actually look at the water. "This is sheer torture," she told me. At the end of most sessions, she'd have a crushing headache caused by the severe stress of being exposed to water for an hour at a time.

I finally felt at wit's end, all but abandoning hope that I could ever really help Mary. Then one afternoon, out of sheer frustration, I decided to try an experiment. Mary and I were sitting in my backyard within sight of the swimming pool. Before long, the close proximity of the water began to affect her. She fidgeted in her chair. She became mildly agitated and eventually very upset. "I feel it in the pit of my stomach," she said. "Every time I look at or think of water I feel it right here in my stomach."

Instantly, I got an idea. Though I have never been formally trained in acupuncture, I was familiar enough with Chinese medicine to understand its theory that energy flows through the body along highways called meridians, which coincide with acupuncture points. When these energy streams become imbalanced, according to this Chinese system, an individual becomes ill. I knew that a spot directly under the eye was the location of an end point to the stomach meridian—and, of course, Mary had said it was her stomach that had developed such a queasy feeling. On a whim, and out of my own desperation, I told Mary, "Tap here." I pointed to a spot just below her eye. "Think about your fear of water, and use two fingers to tap firmly a few times under your eye."

Mary did.

I didn't expect much to happen. But frankly, I was willing to try just about anything. Maybe, just maybe, the rhythmic tapping might balance or unblock her energy flow.

After just two minutes, Mary stopped tapping. She looked at me with amazement in her eyes.

"It's gone!" she exclaimed.

"What's gone?"

"That awful feeling in the pit of my stomach. It's completely gone!"

Completely gone? I looked at Mary skeptically. Frankly, I didn't believe her.

Before I could say another word, Mary sprang from her chair and began running toward the swimming pool. She was smiling, even laughing—and picking up speed. I suddenly realized that if Mary didn't put on the brakes, she'd end up in the pool—and I knew she couldn't swim! At that moment, it was *me* who was feeling terrified!

"Mary, look out!" I shouted as I sprinted after her.

Mary stopped briefly. She turned back to look at me with an enormous grin on her face. "Don't worry, Dr. Callahan, I know I can't swim." (This statement showed that if, in fact, her fear had been eliminated, the treatment hadn't undermined her judgment; she still had a rational respect for the water.) At pool's edge, Mary gazed briefly at her reflection, then bent down and splashed water on her face. I watched in amazement.

"It's gone, Dr. Callahan," she exclaimed. "I'm not afraid anymore."

As you might guess, I was dumbfounded.

That night, Mary conducted the ultimate test of her phobia. Although the ocean had been the focus of so many of her disturbing nightmares, she felt confident enough to confront it directly. In the midst of a rare California thunderstorm, Mary drove to the beach and walked toward the water. Slowly and courageously, she moved forward. The water inched up her body as she waded into the surf. The cold ocean waves splashed on her knees and eventually reached her waist. Through it all, she remained completely free of fear!

Even today, about two decades later, I continue to speak with Mary regularly. Since that brief "tapping" treatment two decades ago, she is still unburdened by any trace of water phobia. Those terrifying nightmares are gone as well.

THE RESEARCH BEGINS

My treatment of Mary had produced absolutely stunning and unexpected results. Frankly, I hardly knew what to make of it for a while. Perhaps it was just a fluke that couldn't be replicated. Or maybe I had stumbled onto something genuine . . . a real breakthrough in the treatment of phobias.

I tried to make sense of what had happened. How could this unusual technique, which was so contrary to all of my training, work so remarkably well and so rapidly? Could the tapping have really influenced the body's energy fields, somehow improving Mary's emotional well-being when years of traditional psychotherapy had failed? Could tapping at a specific point along a meridian have actually stimulated the movement of healing energy throughout Mary's body, as though it were blood flow being reestablished through blocked arteries?

My research began in earnest. I was hopeful that the technique that had worked for Mary would be just as successful with other patients. So I tried it on a few of them, hoping for the best. The results, however, were mostly disappointing. To my dismay, the same approach rarely worked on others. I used it on patients with phobias and many other types of psychological disturbances. But in those early days, before I refined the technique, my success rate was only about 3 percent.

There was a glimmer of hope, however. When the tapping technique *did* work, it was very powerful. Even though only a small minority of patients was helped by this method, I felt that I had made an important breakthrough. So my research continued.

In the ensuing months, I discovered that in some patients, a *series* of points needed to be tapped—and in a specific sequence. In fact, many more people were helped this way, and not just those with phobias. Over time, variations of these tapping sequences clearly produced improvements in many kinds of emotional and psychological distress. I began to recognize that certain emotional disorders required particular treatment formulas, or *algorithms*. Depending on the problem being treated, one series of tapping maneuvers was more effective than the others.

Before long, I had changed forever the way I (and now a growing number of other psychologists and health-care professionals) treated not only phobias, but most other types of psychological problems. Over the years, I have made new discoveries that have refined the program and further enhanced its success. Now, with two decades of research and experience behind me, Thought Field Therapy routinely produces success rates that are unparalleled in the field of psychology. The results with TFT are predictable and measurable, and the technique works in just minutes.

Perhaps most startling, we have even seen the efficacy of TFT in triggering *physiological* changes, producing improvements in *Heart Rate Variability*, and in the process, resolving many health problems, from chronic pain to heart arrhythmias. When physical ailments like these are treated successfully, and we can measure those effects on sophisticated equipment, it confirms in my own mind that TFT is tapping directly into the body's own healing system. It really is a unique, powerful means of healing.

WHAT CAN YOU EXPECT?

If you carefully follow the program in this book, here's what I can promise. The success rates we've achieved with TFT are unprecedented, and there's every reason to expect that you will enjoy success, too. About 75 to 80 percent of patients have been helped with

TFT when using the formulas, or algorithms, you'll find in this book. That's right, 75 to 80 percent of people can expect to have their negative emotions completely resolved. With even more sophisticated refinements of these techniques—through what I call Causal Diagnosis—the success rates have climbed to as high as 98 percent, even with the most difficult cases!

Think of it. Before TFT, my success rate (and those of my colleagues) in curing phobias was only 5 percent using traditional psychotherapy. Now, using the most advanced generations of TFT, the success rate for phobias and other psychological problems has surged to 98 percent! With successes of that magnitude, I strongly believe that TFT is addressing the fundamental cause of emotional distress, and doing so in a way that conventional psychotherapy has never attempted to do.

When I speak about TFT at conferences, most of my fellow psychologists are startled by those high rates of success. After all, they're familiar with their own conventional psychotherapy and what it can accomplish—and their "cure" rates pale in comparison with those of TFT. The kind of success associated with TFT just doesn't occur in mainstream psychotherapy. If you've been treated by a therapist, you know that's true; the number of "cured" patients is embarrassingly small, but it's still the accepted norm. To make matters worse, it typically takes months or years of treatment for traditional practitioners to achieve any success at all—and without any guarantee of a long-term resolution of the problem.

As you read on, you'll see that TFT doesn't fit any of the widely accepted perceptions of what psychotherapy should be. Nor does it duplicate the limited success rates of traditional psychotherapy. Even when patients have exhausted all other approaches, including drugs, before they ever give this new power therapy a try—and thus might be considered "tough cases"—TFT works for them.

You are probably reading this book because you have a particular psychological (or perhaps physical) problem that you hope to eliminate. This book has been designed for you, not only if your emotional upset is considered inappropriate (a phobia, for instance, or an addictive craving for tobacco or alcohol), but also if the psychological turmoil is very appropriate (associated with a traumatic event like a rape or the violent death of a loved one). TFT can eradicate all traces of your emotional distress, defusing the psychological pain and perhaps even healing some of your physical ailments as well.

TFT'S GROWING SUCCESS

Twenty years ago, I was the only therapist practicing Thought Field Therapy. Today, even though most mainstream psychotherapists remain skeptical of TFT—while knowing little about it—this revolutionary approach is being used by many hundreds of psychiatrists, psychologists, physicians, social workers, school counselors, and teachers, not only in the United States, but throughout the world, including in England, France, Germany, Spain, Sweden, Switzerland, Holland, Denmark, Japan, Singapore, Mexico, Brazil, Bolivia, Australia, and Canada. Thought Field Therapy's practitioners were willing to give TFT a try in light of their own dissatisfaction with conventional methods of helping people who come into their offices. Nearly all of them are now duplicating the impressive results I've seen in my own practice. The real beneficiaries, of course, are people like you—many thousands of them. Their lives have been dramatically improved. Despite the lingering skepticism among traditional psychotherapists, I believe your life can change, too.

Not long ago, I treated a thirty-three-year-old woman named Farrah who worked for a major phone company in Singapore. Her boyfriend had walked out on her a month earlier, and she was emotionally crushed. She had been madly in love with him and felt they were soul mates, forever inseparable. In the aftermath of the breakup, Farrah couldn't function. She was well educated and had a very good job, but suddenly found herself overwhelmed with feelings of helplessness and loss of control. She was miserable and refused to acknowledge that this love of her life was gone for good. There were days when she didn't get out of bed. She hardly ate. She numbed her pain with tranquilizers. She stared at her former lover's photograph for hours.

Farrah couldn't understand how a relationship that had been so promising could have ended in so much pain. "I thought I made him so happy," she told me. Then she added, "He hurt me and I'm very bitter."

Crying and shaking uncontrollably, Farrah asked me for help. I told her about TFT, and over the phone we tried the "recipe" that I have formulated for "love pain."

As I guided Farrah through the technique, she tapped specific points on her body, one by one. Within three minutes, the treatment was over—and so was Farrah's emotional pain. She stopped shaking. She became more relaxed. She said that on a 10-point scale, her level of distress had fallen from a 10 to a 3, and then finally to a 1. Her emotional turmoil was gone. Completely gone. Of course, as Farrah said, "I'd still prefer having my boyfriend back." But she felt at peace with the circumstances of her life. Just as important, this dramatic change in her psychological state has persisted. The last time we talked, she had put her broken heart behind her, apparently forever.

Sound too good to be true? Fortunately, you won't have to accept my claims of TFT's effectiveness on faith. This cutting-edge treatment has now been studied intensively and validated repeatedly. And like a Mr. Wizard experiment, you can try it yourself and experience the results. In this book, you'll be guided through a step-by-step self-help program that will allow you to experience the effects of TFT in your own life. You'll find this to be a very accessible program with remarkably simple prescriptions for recovery that have now been tested on thousands of people. These algorithms are easy to learn and simple to use. By carefully following the recommended patterns of tapping and other procedures, you can enjoy treatment success even though you don't have formal training in TFT.

Whether you're hoping for relief from anxiety, trauma, depression, guilt, anger, addictions, fear, or a broken heart, the program in this book can help. And it will do much more than get rid of symptoms; it will eliminate the underlying cause of the emotional pain, almost immediately and usually permanently.

A NEW WAY OF THINKING

This program represents a radical change for psychology, especially clinical psychology. It leaves social science behind and introduces hard science (with laws and strong predictions) into the field of clinical psychology. Emotional problems can now be completely eliminated within minutes. The hard science will be introduced beginning in the next chapter—research, empirical tests, physiological evidence, and repeatable clinical experience confirming TFT's effectiveness.

No longer do you need to settle for traditional psychotherapy that, at best, helps you learn to live with your fears, anxiety, depression, or other problems. Before long, you'll be putting TFT to work in your own life. For most people in emotional and even physical distress, it can provide rapid relief that may have been elusive for years. If you're seeking renewal, quickly and without any risk of side effects, turn the page and get started.

2

TFT BASICS: WHAT IT IS, HOW IT WORKS

NOT LONG AGO, I treated a man named Roy who had just been offered a major promotion at the high-tech firm where he worked. Roy was a forty-two-year-old engineer, handsome and seemingly self-assured. But instead of celebrating the new job opportunity—and the significant pay raise that accompanied it—he went to pieces. "I can't sleep," Roy told me. "I can't concentrate at work. The anxiety is eating me up."

Roy felt so unsettled that you might think he had just been laid off from his job, rather than being offered a promotion and a sizable increase in income. "In my new position, I'll be overseeing an entire division of the company and I'll have much more responsibility," said Roy. Then he paused, sighed heavily, and added, "I know it sounds good, and I should be thrilled. But the whole situation stresses me out. To take the new job, I'll have to move my family to Denver where the corporate headquarters are located. My daughter is in high school, and she'd have to leave her friends behind. I toss and turn at night, just feeling terrible about that."

Then Roy told me about another problem. He knew that the new position would require plenty of public speaking—and that was something he absolutely dreaded. He had always felt uncomfortable at the podium. He'd stammer, becoming tongue-tied and even dizzy. He could feel his heart pounding. Sweat would accumulate on his upper lip. His hands would shake. He sometimes lost his train of thought in front of a group, and it would take him a few moments to collect himself and get back on track.

The more Roy contemplated what the promotion meant, the more he felt like turning it down. "It's so ironic," he said. "I've had my eye on getting this new position for years. And now that it's being handed to me, I feel like running from it."

Roy and I decided to see if Thought Field Therapy could help him get through what he described as a "major life crisis" and a "real turning point" in his life. Together, could we silence his distress so he could make the best decision for himself and his family?

I asked Roy to evaluate the intensity of his distress on a 1-to-10 scale, with 10 representing the worst possible turmoil. He said it was "at least a 9." Then I guided him through a brief Thought Field Therapy "recipe" for anxiety. He tapped a series of specific points on his body. It took only about three minutes.

When Roy was finished, he looked at me with a sense of relief in his eyes. "I really do feel better," he said. "*Much* better. I'm very calm right now. I don't feel any of the distress I did a few minutes ago." It really was astonishing. On the same 10-point scale, Roy said that his anxiety level had fallen dramatically from a 9 to a 1.

A week later, Roy called with more good news: he had formally accepted the promotion and was truly excited about the challenges ahead. He knew that accepting the new job was the best move for both him and his family, despite the adjustments they'd all have to make. He credited TFT with lifting the burden of anxiety from his shoulders, allowing him to make a rational decision about his future.

A SHORTCUT TO WELLNESS

Thought Field Therapy offers simple, effective prescriptions or "recipes" for psychological (and in some cases, even physical) recovery. As Roy discovered, it takes just minutes for this technique to work—not the weeks, months, or years required by traditional psychotherapy.

Most therapists who use my procedures today were understandably quite skeptical before they tried them. After all, what I do is supposed to be impossible. Those who try TFT are surprised to find that it is just as successful as claimed. Nothing in traditional psychotherapy or current psychological theory could have predicted this unprecedented success—nor can either explain it. TFT is truly revolutionary. The terms that you'll become familiar with in these pages—from *perturbation* to *active information* to *Thought Field* itself—are new to psychology, and so is this approach to healing.

Before TFT, when I treated a patient who had just lost a lover, for example, I had him or her relive the most agonizing moments of that broken relationship, session after painful session. The patient often truly suffered through those many hours of therapy. It was retraumatizing—which might have been acceptable if the patient were getting better in the process. But I never felt that I was helping my patient very much to move beyond the pain and resume a normal, productive life.

Before TFT, I would guide my phobic patients through techniques for relaxation, then challenge their false beliefs that were producing the fears. I might hypnotize them, providing them with positive suggestions to combat their phobias. Then I'd directly expose them to the source of their fear—whether it was crowds, insects, or speaking in public—increasing their level of exposure little by little over a period of weeks or months. Clients told me that even if they were finally able to stand on the balcony of a high-rise building or talk in front of a group, they still felt absolutely horrible. Yes, they understood that their fear was irrational—that they shouldn't be afraid—but they couldn't help it. I came to the conclusion that this therapy wasn't eradicating their fear; it was merely persuading them to engage in activities they had absolutely no inclination to do. I certainly wasn't eliminating their fear at its source. And so their suffering persisted.

As you've already learned, TFT doesn't require a lengthy series of uncomfortable treatment sessions that drag on for many months. Nor does it involve the use of any needles or complicated instruments. But it does demand a dramatic shift in thinking about psychological disturbances, their cause and cure. Like other mental health professionals, I was trained to believe that past experiences, various cognitive factors, body chemistry, the nervous system, and the brain itself were the fundamental causes of negative emotions. But in this chapter, you'll learn that this isn't the case at all.

THE EVOLUTION OF TFT

As a child, I suffered from phobias. I vividly remember feeling terrified going through tunnels or looking out from high-rise buildings. Even at that young age, I knew these fears were irrational, although that insight couldn't control my phobias.

Years later, when I was a graduate student in psychology, I would sometimes drive my classmates a little crazy: while they'd seek diversions on Saturday nights, I wanted to discuss and debate what we had studied that week. Somehow, I knew there was more to resolving psychological distress than what I was learning.

Throughout my professional career, I continued to be curious, always searching for answers. I'm reminded of Albert Einstein's response when he was asked how he had made his remarkable discoveries about nature. "By thinking of practically nothing else my whole life," he answered. I was the same way with psychological issues. I was passionate about learning everything I could, exploring new ideas and theories about the origins of psychological illness and its treatment. Nothing interested me more.

Even so, I never felt tied to one particular school of thought in psychology or related fields, and still don't. Over the years, particularly following that initial positive experience with my patient Mary (described in Chapter 1), I focused my research in a number of directions that I thought might help explain what had happened not only with Mary, but also with literally thousands of subsequent patients. As Thought Field Therapy took form, I drew from many disciplines. TFT, in fact, lies at the confluence of quantum physics, biology, meridian (acupuncture) therapy, the Eastern understanding of the mind-body's natural energy system, and, yes, clinical psychology. I had no formal training in acupuncture, but I explored it on my own. I've often said that if I had been formally trained in all of these fields, I probably wouldn't have made the discoveries I did, since I went on this adventure alone, following the path wherever it led. Call it the power of ignorance.

Applied Kinesiology

Along the way, a psychiatrist colleague, Dr. Harvey Ross, introduced me to a muscle-testing procedure that had been developed by Dr. George Goodheart, a chiropractor. Goodheart called his field of study *applied kinesiology*.

In the test, Harvey had me extend my left arm horizontally to the side, and as he tried to push it downward, I was able to resist his effort, feeling quite strong despite the pressure he was applying.

But then he asked me to think of something upsetting. I chose to focus on the image of my home being destroyed by fire. As I did, Harvey pushed again on my outstretched arm using the same force as before. This time, with the negative thought prominent in my mind, I could not keep my arm up. I felt powerless. At that moment, I realized that this was the best demonstration of the mind/body interaction I had ever seen and experienced!

Soon thereafter, I began to ponder the question: If there were a way to maintain my strength while concentrating on a problem, might this indicate that the problem was losing its intensity?

Acupuncture

Acupuncture taps into the body's energy system. This ancient healing system (at least five thousand years old) is based on the premise that by stimulating the flow of energy, the body's own healing network can be activated. Although Thought Field Therapy is much more powerful than acupuncture, producing highly predictable and immediate results, it accesses the same energy system by tapping some of the identical points on the body into which acupuncture needles are inserted. Upon tapping certain points in a particular sequence, psychological problems can be eliminated. As I'll explain shortly, one of the major differences between TFT and the discipline of acupuncture is that my approach also incorporates a technique called *thought tuning* as part of the therapeutic process. With its other unique features, TFT is capable of producing much more powerful healing than acupuncture.

Neurolinguistic Programming

Research in the field of neurolinguistic programming (NLP) has shown the effects that certain eye movements can have on accessing memories and possibly promoting stress reduction and relaxation. All human experience, according to NLP theorists, is encoded in a series of systems that correspond to the sensory network (visual, auditory, kinesthetic) through which one relates to the world. Partially influenced by NLP notions regarding eye movements, as I developed TFT's algorithms, or "recipes," I included some eye movements that contribute to its overall efficacy.

Other Paths of Inquiry

My study of several other disciplines also contributed to the evolution of Thought Field Therapy. For example, as I began to witness the amazing improvements in my patients who used TFT, their "quantum-type leaps" led me to study quantum theory for possible explanations for their dramatic transformations. The writings of quantum theorists like David Bohm helped me understand why TFT was capable of producing such meaningful changes, patient after patient. I was also intrigued by split-brain research suggesting that humming sounds might provide access to the right brain.

Taken together, research in all of these disciplines contributed to and supported what I had been discovering on my own, ultimately leading to the fine-tuning of TFT.

Again, Thought Field Therapy is like no other psychological treatment in terms of the foundation on which it is built—not to mention its record of success. Winston Churchill once said, "People stumble over the truth frequently, but most just pick themselves up and carry on as if nothing happened." Fortunately, when the truth about the causes and treatment of psychological distress crossed my path, I took it to heart. The result: Thought Field Therapy.

Let's get to the specifics of TFT and the science that supports it.

THE THOUGHT FIELD

Einstein demonstrated that everything is energy ($E = mc^2$); Thought Field Therapy is based on the premise that even thought is energy. Perhaps not surprisingly, the energy produced within the brain can be detected and measured with sophisticated tools such as electroencephalography (EEG). Now, for a moment, picture this thought energy as being bound in a field—no more directly observable, but just as real, as a magnetic or gravitational field. Even though you can't see a magnetic or gravitational field, you can experience its effects; the same is true with Thought Fields.

The dictionary defines *field* this way: "a complex of forces that serve as causative agents in human behavior." The Thought Field is the most fundamental concept in TFT. This intangible "structure" or "scaffold" can contain large amounts of information, but in treating psychological distress, we'll concentrate on the information that is generating the negative emotions you are experiencing. When you are terrified of snakes, devastated by a marital breakup, or depressed over the loss of a job, the cause of this disturbance is contained in a Thought Field. Because what you think about during the treatment itself is crucial for the success of this program, I coined the term Thought Field to describe where this critical information is found.

Remember, there is no direct way to observe a Thought Field—or, for that matter, the grief, trauma, or fear you might be feeling. But that does not make it any less real. In the past, physicists couldn't see an electron, but they acknowledged the indirect evidence of its existence.

Some scientists have approached psychological distress in a much different way than I have. They have argued that the fundamental information causing negative emotions is hardwired into the brain, and that the amygdala of the brain is the center of these emotions and cannot be changed. As this theory goes, painful life experiences are permanently embedded in the brain; at best, we can direct attention away from them, or use medications to mask the pain they cause. But there's no way to get rid of them short of some future surgical procedure or some future drug.

My own research—supported by the results of treatment with TFT—seriously undermines this "hardwiring" theory. If hardwiring were true, emotional upsets could not be so rapidly eradicated by TFT. As British biologist Rupert Sheldrake has written, "The memory is no more in the brain than the picture coming from a television studio is in the television receiver." I believe the evidence now shows that we aren't dealing with "hardware" when we're talking about negative emotions; we're dealing with software instead. And this software can be changed very rapidly since it has little inertial mass.

THE ROOT OF THE PROBLEM

So with the concept of the Thought Field in mind, what is the root cause of emotional distress? It is what I call a *perturbation* in a Thought Field. As you may know, in physics and astronomy the term *perturbation* indicates a disturbance in or difference from the norm, and it implies a random quality. But in Thought Field Therapy, the perturbation is hardly random; it is a unique entity that contains *active information* (a quantum physics concept) of a highly specific sort—a subtle, but clearly isolable aspect of the Thought Field—that is responsible for triggering negative emotions. The psychological upset is due *not* to a trauma or the loss of a love, for example. These experiences give rise to the perturbation, but it is the perturbation itself that is responsible for generating, guiding, and controlling all of the fundamental changes within the body—influencing the chemicals, hormones, neural pathways, and cognitive and brain activity—that result in the experience of a specific negative emotion such as fear, anger, or depression. When you're grieving, when you compulsively overeat, or when you're anxious, there is a perturbation in a Thought Field. The perturbation holds the information that governs these and *all* negative or disturbing emotions.

For years, although I knew of the existence of this entity in the Thought Field that created emotional disturbances, I did not know what to call it. I sought a name that would fit the existing knowledge, but would not need to be changed if new information became available. Then the word *perturbation* came to me, and I opened a dictionary to see what it said. One of the dictionary definitions particularly excited me. It defined *perturbation* as "a cause of mental disquietude." When I read that, I knew I'd found the perfect word to describe this entity in the Thought Field. I simply amended the definition slightly, to "*the* cause of mental disquietude."

The perturbation is analogous to the concept of the cell in biology and the atom in chemistry. It is the fundamental unit of causation of all disturbing emotions. Keep in mind that if it were the event itself that caused the emotional turmoil—the loss of a loved one, for example—you couldn't do much to quiet the storm; after all, there is no way to change that past event. Fortunately, perturbations *can* be collapsed and eliminated, thanks to Thought Field Therapy.

TAPPING INTO THE BODY'S ENERGY

I've already mentioned the role of the body's energy system in TFT. This program draws upon Eastern tradition and its understanding of the presence and importance of energy in the body. Let's look at the science behind it a little more closely.

The Chinese use the term *Qi* (pronounced "chee") to describe the vital life energy. When the flow of this energy becomes blocked or imbalanced, according to the Chinese, it can trigger physical illnesses. Just as acupuncturists have developed ways to eliminate pain and promote physical healing by manipulating energy flows along a network of so-called meridians, or pathways, throughout the body, I have shown that these energy pathways can be accessed in order to heal emotional distress.

The body's energy system has not been ignored by Western researchers, who have applied hard science to this ancient knowledge. As far back as the 1940s, Harold Saxon Burr of Yale University hypothesized that an internal energy system was key to humans and all living things. Robert O. Becker, M.D., an orthopedic surgeon, used electromagnetic energy fields to stimulate the natural healing of broken bones and found that electromagnetic fields could be used to help regenerate amputated limbs in frogs.

Some of the most intriguing research was conducted by Dr. Bjorn Nordenstrom, a prominent Swedish scientist and radiologist and former president of the Nobel prize nominating committee. In studies spanning two decades, he actually documented the existence of these electrical circuits in the body. Nordenstrom's interest in this area started when he observed a halo around malignant lung tumors and began looking for an explanation for this phenomenon. He identified a circulatory energy system in the body, which he felt was just as significant to physical well-being as the blood circulatory system. He demonstrated that electric circuits are carried by the interstitial spaces (the spaces between cells) and the blood vessels, and he believed that disruptions in the human energy system may play a role in the development of diseases as serious as cancer. He began cutting-edge research in which patients with metastatic cancer who were believed to be terminal were treated with applications of electrical currents—with promising results. Another researcher, French biochemist Jacques Hauton, wrote that Nordenstrom's findings led him to conclude that the electrical system "is not only as complex as the circulation of blood, but it also . . . intervenes in all physiological activity."

In 1995, Pierre de Vernejoul provided concrete evidence that the meridian network does exist. He and his team of investigators injected nonharmful radioactive technetium 99m into the arms and legs of human volunteers at the sites of commonly used acupuncture points along the meridian system. Then they used gamma-camera imaging to track the flow of this injected material. They found that the radioactive isotope traveled specifically along the meridian pathways that the Chinese had identified thousands of years ago. By contrast, when the substance was injected randomly elsewhere in the body, it did not move along any specific internal pathway. The bottom line: the meridian system is an actual, clearly defined network—the same one the Chinese have been using for millennia.

Thus, the energy system used in Thought Field Therapy is genuine, not some mystical notion. Every perturbation in the Thought Field is associated with a specific energy meridian. My own research has shown that the meridian system is a governing force in controlling and healing the disturbing emotions. Best of all, this system can be accessed by TFT. This is true whether the psychological problem is anxiety, trauma, addictions, panic attacks, phobias, anxiety, anger, jealousy, or depression. More recently, we've learned that TFT seems capable of producing physical healing as well. By tapping on specific points along the body's energy meridians, rebalancing and healing can take place at the most fundamental level, weakening and eliminating the underlying negative emotion or physical ailment. As the stimulation from this tapping influences the internal electromagnetic energy, it has a direct effect on the Thought Field and the perturbation associated with the problem being treated.

As you learn the self-administered algorithms that are key to Thought Field Therapy, you will tap on points along these energy meridians that have been chosen specifically for the particular emotional (or physical) distress you're having, and sequenced in a specific way, like the order of a combination lock. If the sequence is wrong or the points are inappropriate, the lock won't open; but if they are correct, healing will occur, rapidly and usually permanently. The "recipe" for each problem has been initially validated on hundreds and, in some cases, even thousands of people and is now widely accepted as an algorithm. Each can achieve predictable results in patient after patient.

HEALING WITH ALGORITHMS

If you've tried traditional psychotherapy to treat your emotional problems, a healing algorithm may be a difficult concept to grasp.

Many of my patients initially respond this way—until they try it. Again, the key element of each algorithm is tapping particular points on the body, selected from among twelve major points located along the energy meridians. Remember, these brief recipes are different for each emotional disorder—that is, there is a distinct tapping sequence for resolving phobias, another one for "love pain," and so on. In that sense, each algorithm is like a custom-tailored suit rather than one bought off the rack; it is designed specifically for a particular type of psychological distress. The specificity of TFT opens the door to recovery time after time. The healing energy is already contained within the body, just waiting to be accessed by the correct algorithm that can release it and stimulate a full recovery.

Keep in mind that these targeted recipes were not created by intuition or a trial-and-error process. They have grown out of careful evaluation of the scientific evidence—my own and that of others. In recent years, they have been refined through a complex procedure called Causal Diagnosis, which has become an integral part of TFT, and which I'll discuss later. It is a method by which we can determine with precision the "code" responsible for producing and healing a particular psychological problem. Remember, every algorithm—in fact, each portion of every algorithm—has been tested before being incorporated into the healing technique. At times, I've felt something like Thomas Edison when he tried many different filaments before finding the one that worked. In TFT, the final arbiter has been the reality of whether patients get better. And ultimately, nearly all of them do.

TUNING THE THOUGHT FIELD

As you'll discover, you need more than the right algorithm for TFT to work. An equally crucial part of the therapy involves "tuning the Thought Field"—that is, thinking about your emotional problem as you are treating it. Remember, the perturbation is what you are targeting, and since it is contained in the Thought Field, you need to access it by thinking about the psychological upset in your life.

To tune a Thought Field, you don't have to concentrate. The process simply involves intentionally thinking about the problem that is causing you so much distress. As you proceed through the algorithm, you'll need to focus your attention on the person, the event, the situation, or whatever else is associated with your emotional upset, but it won't take any unusual effort.

Tuning the Thought Field may actually upset you; in fact, it probably will. If you're grieving over the death of a close friend, for example, or if you're absolutely petrified of dogs, shifting all of your attention to this problem or situation will understandably make you sad, afraid, upset, or distressed. As that happens, a cascade of physiological activity—such as the release of chemicals associated with emotions—will be triggered. These uncomfortable feelings and experiences can be strong enough to leave you wondering (albeit briefly) whether this is all worth it. But consider it a short-term "sacrifice" worth making. After all, this kind of psychological and physiological response indicates that one or more powerful perturbations are present in that Thought Field and need to be eliminated. While you may be feeling distressed and agitated for a few minutes as you tune the Thought Field and begin to implement the algorithm, the payoff is that the emotional problem should literally disappear in minutes. The therapy wouldn't be effective if you didn't think about the problem that is causing so much pain. You can't treat a Thought Field unless it's tuned.

No doubt this is very different from any other treatment you're familiar with. When you undergo acupuncture, for example, "thought tuning" is not required. Nor is it required by mainstream physicians or chiropractors. These practitioners don't care what you're thinking about when you're under their care. Your dentist doesn't ask you to concentrate on your molars while he or she is filling a cavity; your teeth aren't going to respond to the treatment any differently, no matter what's on your mind. In these cases, what you're thinking about is irrelevant. At times, I've challenged skeptics to test this notion by having patients use the algorithms when they *aren't* tuning the Thought Field—and then to repeat the process while tuning. What a difference!

As you tune the Thought Field while stimulating the appropriate meridians, you can literally eliminate the negative emotion by collapsing the perturbation that is the source of the psychological turmoil—and you can do it within minutes. The fear of heights that may have plagued you for decades . . . the distress over the death of a parent years earlier . . . all of that emotional upset will be gone, usually for good.

After successful TFT treatment, you will notice that you are no longer distressed. Some people erroneously believe that this is because they simply aren't thinking of the problem anymore. This is a typical reaction, but you should know that it is impossible to say the words "I cannot think about the problem" without in fact thinking about it. After the TFT treatment, you no longer can get upset while thinking about the problem. That's because the problem is gone.

THE ISOLABLE NATURE OF PERTURBATIONS

One of the most interesting aspects of this process is that the perturbation is *isolable*. I use that term because the algorithm will collapse the perturbation in the problem Thought Field, but in doing so, it won't affect the Thought Field in any other way. If you were in an automobile accident in which a loved one was seriously injured, for example, you'd still recall the incident in detail. Any profound life experience will always be with you. But thanks to TFT, its emotional charge will be defused. It will no longer trigger excruciating, debilitating distress. When you think about the event, the details might even become clearer once the disruptive emotions are eliminated. Nevertheless, there will be no discomfort, no pain.

Again, it is not the automobile accident itself that causes the emotional upset but the perturbation. Fortunately, the perturbation is automatically isolated from the rest of the Thought Field and can be eliminated. Everything else in that Thought Field will remain just as it was. After the treatment, when you think about the event that had triggered such psychological upset just minutes earlier, it will cause no such emotional response. If you had been having nightmares associated with the emotional problem, they should disappear as well. Since the perturbation is gone, so are all remnants of the psychological turmoil associated with it.

Of course, most traditional psychotherapists will tell you that when you lose a loved one, for example, you should go through a long grieving process. They may even say that feeling that grief is necessary, even desirable. But I've always thought this was a rationalization. They simply don't know how to get rid of the pain, so they tell patients, "The pain you're feeling is normal and healthy."

As a family physician who was mourning the death of a loved one said, "The most compassionate advice I get from friends and professional colleagues who are unfamiliar with TFT [is] to go into my pain, feel it, and that it will take a year. Well, I found that it doesn't take a year. It can take only minutes, in fact."

If people want to suffer, well, that's their choice. But I can help them eradicate those negative emotions for good!

One of my earliest patients was a woman named Julia. She was in her late thirties and had been diagnosed with terminal cancer. Of course, her grim prognosis was a devastating blow to her and her family. She had traveled to California from her home in Chicago to get a second opinion, which turned out to be no more encouraging than the original one: she was given less than a year to live.

Julia was referred to me by her physician in hopes that I could help her deal with the emotional devastation she was feeling. She had been crying uncontrollably during most of her waking hours. She experienced panic attacks throughout the day. Julia's reaction to her uncertain future was completely understandable and even appropriate. I never considered her to have a psychological problem; after all, who wouldn't react to a situation like hers with fear and distress? So treating her was completely different than treating someone with, say, a fear of spiders, which is an *inappropriate* response to a harmless bug. Still, the emotional devastation that kept Julia on the brink of hysteria was making it impossible for her to function and enjoy the remaining time she had with her husband and young children.

I treated Julia with Thought Field Therapy. There was no real need to ask her to tune the Thought Field; she could think of nothing else. Nevertheless, I asked her to focus upon the terrible disease that threatened her life. Then I guided her through the rest of the therapy.

Within minutes, Julia said she felt like a different person. Her cancer had not been affected by Thought Field Therapy. But after the treatment, when I asked her to think about her illness and how it might end her life prematurely, she did not become upset. She began talking about the disease matter-of-factly, free of the emotional charge that had been there minutes earlier. To confirm in my own mind that I hadn't merely distracted Julia from her illness, I asked her to explain what she was feeling about the ominous reality of her life circumstances. "Well," she said, "I don't like it at all, that's for sure. But my upset and fear seem to be gone. I feel surprisingly strong right now in the face of this terrible diagnosis." Almost instantly, her outlook on life was dramatically altered. Of course, she would have preferred that her circumstances were very different. But the emotional anguish that had overwhelmed her was gone.

What had happened to Julia? By now, you should know the answer. Thanks to TFT, the perturbation in the treated Thought Field had been eliminated; the powerful emotions that had so incapacitated her had collapsed.

Consider this fact: when the Thought Field is tuned before therapy, it creates enormous distress; after treatment, the same attuned Thought Field produces no upset. I take this as clear evidence that something in the Thought Field has changed as a result of the treatment. Now, thanks to the technology of *Heart Rate Variability* (which I'll discuss in Chapter 3), we are able to concretely measure the transformation that is occurring in the autonomic nervous system as a result of TFT. Real, verifiable, physiological and emotional changes take place. We are addressing the fundamental cause of an individual's upset—the perturbation—and eliminating or removing it during therapy. There is no trace of the distress left. It is a predictable process, occurring in patient after patient.

When I have followed up with patients like Julia, in some cases over many years, the benefits of the treatment typically persist. In fact, the troubling thoughts have completely lost their ability to trigger psychological turmoil. Even if you try to get back in touch with all that emotional upset, you won't be able to.

Remember, TFT won't change the reality of the event that might be causing your distress. For example, it won't bring back the spouse who abandoned you and make everything right again. Or if your child has died, you will have to live with that reality for the rest of your life; there is no way to erase that tragedy. But TFT *will* eliminate the hurt and the pain that have surrounded that terrible event for so long. It will allow you to begin leading and even enjoying your life again.

THE POWER OF TFT

Can Thought Field Therapy really work for you? You will soon find out. As I noted in Chapter 1, the algorithms consistently work for 75 to 80 percent of people—a success rate many, many times greater than traditional psychotherapy. One of the most amazing features of TFT is that because it produces results so quickly, you'll know almost instantly whether the treatment has been successful.

Over the years, the rapidity with which this therapy works has also provided me with wonderful opportunities to refine the treatment. When I was a traditional practitioner, I was like other therapists, engaged in something like throwing darts at a dartboard but never really seeing where they landed. No wonder it is so hard for mainstream psychotherapists to truly help anyone. But with TFT, if I'm not on target, I know immediately. When I'm not hitting the bull's-eye, I can make adjustments and refinements that, over time, have raised the success rate of TFT to unprecedented levels.

Today, Thought Field Therapy works for people of all ages, across all social and cultural lines, and even for the most severe problems (it has also been effective in dogs, cats, and horses!). One of my patients—I'll call her Linda—had experienced one of the most horrible traumas imaginable. She had been repeatedly and brutally raped by four gang members who had broken into her apartment and held her prisoner for a week while they took turns sexually assaulting her. When she came to see me, she was still haunted and constantly distressed by this monstrous event in her life, even though it had happened ten years earlier. Over that time, she had been unable to date or even be alone with a man. She was a divorcée, and her son had been four years old when the rape occurred. Linda said the worst part of that horrific week was that her child was in the apartment with her when the rape happened, and the intruders repeatedly threatened to kill both her and the terrified boy.

Linda's reaction to what had happened was thoroughly appropriate. Who wouldn't be traumatized by such a horrible experience? This was a real-life event, not an irrational fear. Despite the enormity of her emotional distress, could she be helped to move beyond it? Could she lead a normal life again? Most mental health professionals would answer these questions negatively, insisting that this trauma would haunt her forever. I knew that Linda's case would be a real test of Thought Field Therapy.

Like most TFT treatments, Linda's took only about five minutes. And sure enough, Linda seemed immediately relieved. Her level of distress had plummeted from a 10 to a 1 (on a 10-point scale). Although the horrible reality of the rape could not be erased, all traces of her emotional turmoil were gone. I continued to follow her for two years. Her upset never returned. The nightmares vanished for good. And, by the way, after I treated her son as well, he had no apparent emotional upset remaining.

ARE YOU A SKEPTIC?

To many people, particularly those trained in conventional psychology, Thought Field Therapy seems, at best, peculiar. Because of their background and education, they can't believe TFT could possibly work. For them, it is just not a reasonable way to approach emotional problems. But, of course, once they observe (and sometimes personally experience) the results, their interest is piqued. Even for the skeptics, it is hard to deny the fact that this is the most powerful and effective therapy now available.

When I describe Thought Field Therapy to my own trainees, I often tell them that when TFT was being developed, I studied nature firsthand—and TFT revealed itself to me. I uncovered the control system for the emotions, related intimately to the meridians, that nature itself has created for renewal and healing. TFT clearly works, whether the problem at hand is anger, anxiety, depression, jealousy, or any other negative emotion. By activating the energy meridian system with the correct encodings, perturbations in the Thought Field can be collapsed, eliminating the psychological problem at the deepest level.

Remarkably, even if you're still a little skeptical right now, even if you're questioning whether the system in this book can really help, TFT can still work for you. You don't have to have faith that the treatment will succeed for it to be effective. It is not necessary that you understand or even accept the science behind it. Like an effective antibiotic, it will work whether or not you believe it will.

Psychologist Gale L. Joslin, Ph.D., tells the story of strolling with a friend along the boardwalk at Venice Beach in Los Angeles and describing the anxiety he was feeling about a psychopharmacology exam that both were going to take the following day. As they walked, the friend told Gale about a therapeutic technique he had just learned—Thought Field Therapy—that could help anxiety and many other psychological problems, and he suggested that Gale try it.

Gale agreed, and for the next couple minutes, his friend led him through a TFT algorithm. He instructed Gale to tap near the eyebrow, under the eye, under the arm, and on the chest, and to add other elements as well (including counting and humming). As Gale later said, "By this time, I knew my friend was crazy! But, because he is my best friend, I humored him and did as he asked."

Gale quickly recognized, however, that something quite remarkable was happening. Before the treatment began, he had rated his anxiety as a 10 on the Subjective Units of Distress scale—that is, it couldn't go any higher. But after the treatment, the anxiety had disappeared. Gale even tried to get the anxiety back, but he couldn't. It was gone.

The following day, Gale took the exam without experiencing even a trace of anxiety. He completed the three-hour test in just one hour and scored very well. He is now a diplomate in psychopharmacology and a leading practitioner of TFT. With twenty years in practice, Gale has written, "I have never seen anything like TFT for effectiveness. What might have taken months or years of treatment now takes one or two sessions for most cases."

Over the years, I've found that one of the best ways to silence skepticism is to treat people with the TFT algorithms in a public setting, including on television shows. I've explained to TV producers that I don't want to merely talk about TFT on their programs; it is much more valuable to viewers to see the technique being used with volunteers—the more severe and long-lasting the psychological problems, the better. So, for example, for one TV program shot on location at the Bonaventure Hotel in Los Angeles, three people with a fear of heights and enclosed spaces were treated with TFT. Then, without a trace of anxiety, these volunteers rode the hotel's outside glass elevators, which would have been a veritable nightmare for them before their acrophobia and claustrophobia were cured.

In TV studios, I have treated people who were afraid of snakes, needles, spiders, rats, and ladders, among other things. When I appeared on a morning TV talk show with Regis Philbin, where I was discussing an earlier book I had written, Regis said, "The test is this: either the guy's cure works or it doesn't. Rarely do you get a chance to test these authors who come through here with their books." Of course, it was possible for me to fail on live television. But, overall, I've had a success rate of over 90 percent on television—which helped silence many skeptics.

When people ask, "What's the evidence that TFT works?" I often refer them to the scientific studies that support it and urge them to try it (see Chapter 3). But much more often, here's how I quiet their doubts: I treat them. TFT works even in the face of skepticism on the part of both the patient *and* the therapist. The treatment is so powerful that it is capable of overriding whatever negative influence the skepticism may carry.

In the chapters that follow, you'll find just how rapidly Thought Field Therapy can work for you. Remember, although the system in this book took many years to develop and refine, it can produce results in minutes. By my definition, a complex case is one in which the psychological problem hasn't been resolved in five minutes. Fortunately, relatively few cases are complex.

Not long ago, I treated a patient named Nancy who had struggled with an anxiety disorder for decades. For nearly twenty of those years, she had been seeing a psychotherapist. That's right, almost twenty years—and with nothing to show for it in terms of improvement (although she did have an enormous stack of bills from her therapist that could produce high anxiety in just about anyone!).

"My doctor really hasn't done much to help me," Nancy told me. "I'm no better than I was twenty years ago."

"So why have you gone to him for so long?" I asked.

She paused for a moment, contemplating the question. Then she responded, "I like having someone to tell my problems to."

Maybe so. But, as I asked Nancy, "Why don't you just find a friend instead?"

I've heard psychotherapy referred to as "the purchase of friendship." Maybe it has served a useful purpose in that way. However, a friend, a clergyman, or even a bartender might be able to offer the same listening service for a lot less money. In any case, by the time Nancy left my office, the anxiety disorder was no longer among her problems.

The reason conventional psychotherapy has such a poor track record is that it has been playing the "wrong game." The problem is not fundamentally in the cognitive system, in past experience, or in the brain or nervous system. It is in the Thought Field.

3

THE SCIENCE BEHIND TFT

THOUGHT FIELD THERAPY is very counterintuitive. In a psychotherapeutic tradition that emphasizes talk therapy and/or drugs to treat emotional problems, what could be more peculiar than accessing energy systems by tapping specific points on the body—and, in the process, providing healing in just minutes?

As you'll see, in the following pages there's plenty of evidence supporting the effectiveness of TFT. And it not only works in the hands of the professionals who are using it with their own clients and students, but also by lay people like you who have learned the TFT algorithms.

THE WEIGHT OF THE EVIDENCE

In addition to my own clinical research into Thought Field Therapy, which now spans two decades, investigators in all parts of the world have put TFT to the test. They are serious scientists who followed the research where it took them—and were often startled by what they uncovered. These studies can be important in building your own confidence in TFT. Let's review some of this research.

Figley/Carbonell Studies

Charles Figley, Ph.D., and Joyce L. Carbonell, Ph.D., psychologists at Florida State University, have conducted several studies of TFT. In one of them, called a systematic clinical demonstration (SCD) study, they compared the effectiveness of four relatively new therapies—Thought Field Therapy, eye movement desensitization and reprocessing (EMDR), visual kinesthetic dissociation, and traumatic incident reduction—in 156 patients who had suffered a trauma or had a phobia. They used a number of measures, including the Subjective Units of Distress (SUD) scale, to evaluate the effectiveness of the techniques. On the SUD scale, 10 is the worst emotional disturbance possible, and 1 corresponds to a complete absence of distress or pain (I'll discuss the SUD again in Chapter 4).

In this clinical study, Drs. Figley and Carbonell found that all four forms of these newer therapies were helpful. However, the patients using TFT showed significantly more improvement than those using any of the other treatments. Also, the improvements associated with TFT not only occurred in the shortest period of time, but were enduring, continuing throughout the ensuing six months. The researchers concluded that people using TFT "achieved rapid relief from their emotional distress and the treatment appears to be permanent."

Later, Dr. Carbonell and one of her students, Neta Mappa, conducted an experiment as a follow-up to the original Figley/Carbonell research. The 156 college students who signed up for the new study all said they had a fear of heights (or acrophobia).

A screening measure, the Cohn Acrophobia Questionnaire, was used to evaluate their phobia, and forty-nine of them scored high enough on the scale to be considered acrophobic. These forty-nine volunteers were then given a behavioral test in which they were asked to climb a four-foot ladder. As Dr. Carbonell wrote, "We hoped that the ladder was of sufficient height to provoke an acrophobic response, but not so high as to put the subject at physical risk." As each individual climbed the ladder, he or she was asked to rate the fear on every step, using the SUD scale. The subjects were told that they could stop climbing the ladder at any time.

Once this phase of the study was completed, the students were taken to another room, where an investigator asked them to think of anxiety-producing circumstances related to heights, and then to rate their anxiety on a 0-to-10 scale (this study employed an 11-point SUD scale). Next, the subjects were randomly assigned to proceed through either the TFT algorithm for phobias or a placebo TFT (consisting of tapping on parts of the body not used in TFT algorithms). Once the treatment was completed, the students were told again to rate themselves on the SUD scale. If the rating was not zero, the treatment was repeated one additional time. Finally, the subjects returned to the ladder and were asked to climb it, providing the investigators with a SUD score every step of the way.

When Carbonell and Mappa evaluated their data, it showed that there were no differences in pretherapy measurements between the TFT and the placebo groups. After treatment, however, the differences were significant. Both groups got somewhat better, but the individuals undergoing TFT experienced significantly more improvement when compared with the placebo group. According to Carbonell, "Those who were treated with TFT had less anxiety than those who received the placebo. . . . The clinical study and the experimental study, taken together, provide support for TFT."

Stephen Daniel Study

After Stephen Daniel, Ph.D., was trained in advanced TFT (called Voice Technology), he decided to evaluate the effectiveness of the technique in a clinical study. His subjects were a particularly challenging group to treat—214 other therapists, all of whom had psychological difficulties that they wanted to resolve. These professionals had problems that included panic attacks, depression, addictive cravings, obsessive-compulsive disorder, and trauma and post-trauma disorders. Some also had physical ailments such as chronic pain, migraines, fibromyalgia, tinnitus, chronic cough, asthma attacks, hypertension, insomnia, and poor libido. None had been helped by other forms of treatment.

The level of each patient's emotional distress was evaluated on the SUD scale. Then each individual underwent a single treatment of TFT, using a sophisticated form of the technique called Voice Technology; the average time for each treatment was just under five minutes. After this one brief therapeutic session, the results were quite remarkable: SUD ratings declined significantly from an initial average of 7.74 down to an average of 1.11. In follow-up contact with the subjects, most reported maintaining their improvements. These results were published in November 1998.

Radio Studies

Some of the research into Thought Field Therapy has been in less formal settings, but the results have been no less impressive. In the mid-1980s, I appeared on nearly two dozen radio shows discussing TFT. To demonstrate how effective the technique could be, and how easy it is to use, I tested it on callers who had phobias. On the air, I invited calls from listeners who would become distressed just by thinking about the source of their fear (most people with phobias fall into this category). As listeners phoned in, I led each person through a treatment based on Voice Technology that involved tapping on particular points on the body in a specific order. Each treatment took less than five minutes (which included the time spent explaining this unfamiliar therapy to each caller). I calculated the effectiveness of the treatment by asking the volunteers to evaluate the intensity of their distress before and after the treatment, using the 10-point SUD scale.

I kept careful records and audiotapes of each of these treatments administered on the radio. At the end, I had data on sixty-eight callers, and I turned it over to an independent evaluator, who tabulated and analyzed the results. The findings, which appear in the table on the following page, were startling. A "successful" treatment was defined as a decrease of two or more points on the SUD scale; using that criterion, 97 percent of the volunteers were considered to have been successfully treated. As the table indicates, the average decline in the SUD rating exceeded six points—a dramatic 76 percent drop!

Why did I choose radio programs to put TFT to the test? On the one hand, it wasn't a perfect forum for treating emotional problems. On the other, I felt the setting was ideal for minimizing the effects of positive expectations, which are often present when a patient comes to a therapist's office and pays for treatment. Also, by performing the technique so publicly, the results—whether good or bad—would be evident to everyone, thus reducing any skepticism that is sometimes associated with claims made by psychologists on research carried out in the privacy of their offices or laboratories.

As impressive as my own results were, could they be replicated? Ten years after my study, a trainee conducted research almost identical to mine. He, too, treated people on live radio shows (when he reached 68 callers—the same number as in my study—he stopped). They had a wide range of psychological disturbances, not only phobias but also anxiety, addictive cravings, guilt, obsessive-compulsive disorders, and marital problems. As part of this study, the trainee used an advanced TFT technique (Voice Technology), as I had done, to diagnose the specific problem of each caller, and then he based his TFT treatment on those findings.

Using the SUD rating instrument (this second study employed an 11-point scale, from 0 to 10), 97 percent of the callers were considered successfully treated with TFT. Amazingly, this success was identical to what I had achieved a decade earlier. As the chart below shows, the average pre- and post-therapy SUD score had declined significantly. Again, these results were attained rapidly, in an average of about six minutes!

THE RADIO STUDIES: RESULTS

	Callahan (1985–1986)	Trainee (1995–1996)
Number of radio shows	23	36
Number of patients treated	68	68
Successfully treated	66	66
Unsuccessfully treated	2	2
Success rate	97%	97%
Pretherapy: average distress/anxiety level (SUD)	8.35 *(10-point scale)*	8.19 *(11-point scale)*
Post-therapy: average distress/anxiety level (SUD)	2.01 *(1 = best possible)*	1.58 *(0 = best possible)*
Average improvement in distress/anxiety level (SUD)	6.34	6.61
Average time (includes all talk and explanation to the end of treatment)	4.34 minutes	6.04 minutes

In my own study, a separate analysis focused on those callers whose complaint had been a fear of public speaking. Of course, the mere act of talking on live radio would be terrifying for someone frightened of speaking in public. So for these individuals, treatment with TFT was performed at precisely the moment in which they were being exposed directly to their phobia. Their SUD ratings would be a realistic evaluation of TFT's effectiveness.

What were those results? The data showed that among the eleven volunteers in this study with a public-speaking phobia, *all* of them improved after TFT. Overall, their average SUD score declined from 8.8 prior to treatment to 1.9 after treatment.

Other Studies

Serious research into TFT is moving ahead at an accelerated pace. Let me briefly relate the findings of two additional studies.

In the first, Robert L. Bray, Ph.D., LCSW, Adjunct Professor of Social Work at San Diego State University, and Crystal Folkes, M.S., used TFT to treat immigrants and refugees experiencing post-traumatic stress symptoms. The specific traumatic events in their lives ranged from single acts of psychological threat to multiple incidents of violence and torture.

Before the TFT treatments began, the subjects completed psychological testing that evaluated their trauma-related symptoms. Then a team of counseling interns trained in the TFT algorithms administered the therapy, which was overseen by a supervisor. Among the thirty-four subjects who were guided through an algorithm, and who also completed the pretest (and later a post-test), there was an average post-therapy decline of almost 40 percent in their symptoms. Among a subgroup of twenty-nine individuals whose pretest scores clearly indicated a diagnosis of post-traumatic stress disorder (PTSD), 62 percent (or eighteen people) had post-test scores showing so much improvement that they no longer met the diagnostic criteria for PTSD. Ultimately, 79 percent of these twenty-nine patients reported that they had experienced significant declines in the frequency of symptoms associated with post-traumatic stress.

In the second study, Ian Graham of the United Kingdom used one of the advanced TFT techniques called Causal Diagnosis to treat 177 people who were experiencing a variety of psychological problems. All but eleven of these subjects responded positively to the treatment, thus producing improvement in 94 percent of individuals. The average SUD score declined dramatically, from a pretreatment level of 8.29 to a post-treatment level of 2.17.

As encouraging as formal studies have been, perhaps the strongest scientific validation of TFT is simply how predictably people like you experience improvements and cures. The algorithms in this book will let you test the claims for yourself, without million-dollar studies and control groups. The impressive findings are easily reproducible by practically everyone. With the levels of success we've achieved, we have elevated psychotherapy into the cherished domain of hard science.

TFT AND YOUR PHYSICAL HEALTH

"Take two aspirin and call me in the morning."

That familiar advice from your physician may be replaced soon with a different kind of recommendation: "Try a TFT algorithm and call me in the morning."

There's really nothing improbable about that scenario. In fact, a current area of intensive research into Thought Field Therapy is its effects on *physiological* ailments. Of course, TFT was originally developed to treat emotional disturbances, where its benefits are now proven. But now it is increasingly clear that the power of this therapeutic technique can be extended to many physical disorders as well. That's right—if you have heart arrhythmias, migraines, fibromyalgia, or asthma attacks, among other ailments, TFT may be able to help.

Years ago, when I first began working with Thought Field Therapy for psychological distress, I began noting some obvious physical changes in patients undergoing TFT. For example, when they were treated successfully, I observed that the coloring would return to their face, giving them a much healthier appearance. To me, this was clear evidence that TFT was having biological as well as psychological effects. The explanation for this change in coloring probably lies with an accelerated delivery of oxygen throughout the body related to TFT's established ability to reduce the clumping of red blood cells in ways that interfere with the transport of oxygen.

To illustrate this point, let me describe an early incident involving a technician who routinely performed laboratory tests that evaluated this clumping of red blood cells. She had the flu the day I met with her. Her complexion was gray, and she complained of feeling absolutely dreadful. I suggested that we try an experiment to see if I could help her feel a little better. I began by asking her to rate how she felt on a 10-point scale, with 10 being as bad as a person can possibly feel. She didn't hesitate. "Believe me," she exclaimed, "I'm a 10, but that's only because 10 is as high as the scale goes!" Next, at my request, she drew a small sample of her own blood and placed a few drops under the microscope. We were able to look at it together on a television monitor. Clearly, the red blood cells were clustered. She said the sample showed "100 percent rouleaux"—that is, the amount of red cell clumping was at its highest possible (and most undesirable) level.

At that point, I treated the technician with TFT. It took just a few minutes. Immediately, some coloring returned to her face. As that happened, she reported feeling somewhat better, perhaps down to a 7 on the 10-point scale. Then she drew another small blood sample. Under the microscope, the amount of clumping had clearly declined to 70 percent!

We proceeded with another TFT treatment. As we did, the coloring continued to return to her face. At the same time, the flu symptoms appeared to subside even further. She rated her sense of well-being again, finally placing it at a 1. Her last blood sample showed *no* trace of rouleaux, or red blood cell clumping (see Figure 3.1). The total time for the TFT treatments and the blood tests was about eight minutes.

"I've never seen rouleaux changes like this," she exclaimed. "Sometimes I've seen these changes over a period of months with medical or chiropractic treatment—but never immediately. Never!"

I began to ponder the implications of what I had just witnessed. If TFT could produce changes within the bloodstream, what other physical effects were occurring?

Not long thereafter, I was invited to discuss TFT on a television talk show. While backstage, waiting to go on the air, I sat in the green room next to a friend of the show's host. This middle-

FIGURE 3.1: ROULEAUX (UNDER THE MICROSCOPE) BEFORE AND AFTER TFT TREATMENTS

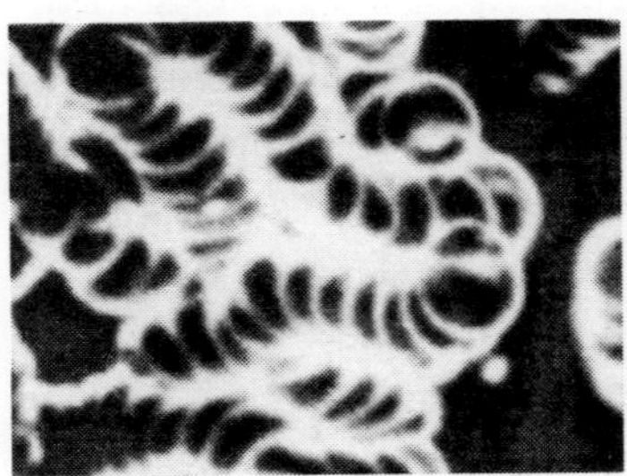

Rouleaux rated at 100 percent by lab technician. Patient totally exhausted, felt she was getting the flu. Rated 10 on the fatigue scale.

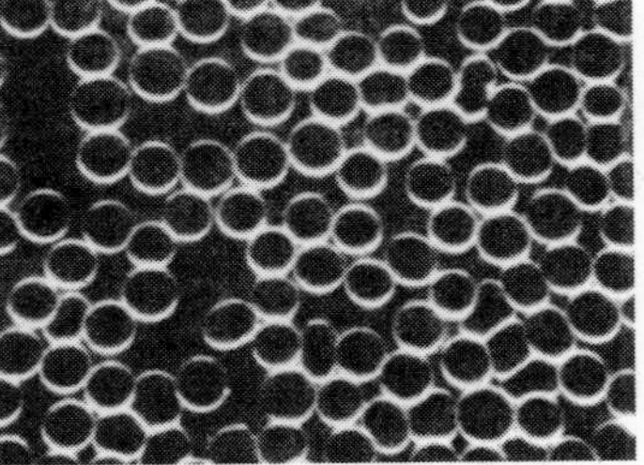

Ten minutes later, after Callahan treatment. Rouleaux rated at 0 percent. Patient felt great, no more flu symptoms. Rated 1 on the fatigue scale.

aged man told me that his arm had been crushed in a serious automobile accident ten years earlier. "I've been in horrible pain ever since," he said. "I've taken painkillers by the handful. I've tried nerve blocks. Nothing has helped. Sometimes I'm in so much agony that it's hard to even face the day."

You could feel the misery coming through his voice. I still had a few minutes until I was scheduled to go before the cameras, and I figured I had nothing to lose. "Let's try something," I told him. I guided him through a TFT algorithm. You could see the skepticism in his eyes when we began, but he was still willing to see what might happen. Within minutes, that skepticism had vanished along with his discomfort. For the first time in years, he said, his pain was gone. "This is amazing," he told me. "My doctor won't believe it."

Since then, I have helped many people with physical complaints by using TFT. A nurse in Toronto suffering from chronic fatigue syndrome used the sequence of tapping movements, and in minutes, she reported that her exhaustion was gone. A woman with metastasized liver cancer had been suffering with intractable pain that her doctors couldn't relieve with analgesic drugs or any other treatment; it seemed like TFT was at least worth a try. It worked remarkably well, eliminating nearly all of her pain.

How does Thought Field Therapy resolve persistent pain, chronic fatigue, or any other physical ailment? In the same way it eliminates emotional problems. It activates the body's healing system and, as we'll discuss below, directly influences the autonomic nervous system.

I'm also convinced that no technique has the power to reduce stress more than TFT does—and as you probably know, stress can have a devastating effect on physical health. If you always feel taxed to the limit, if your life seems out of balance, and if the pressures of life are wearing you down and burning you out, you may be more susceptible to heart disease, high blood pressure, stroke, and cancer—in other words, the major health problems of modern civilization. Fortunately, TFT can now help.

HEART RATE VARIABILITY: MEASURING THE POWER OF TFT

The most dramatic and objective evidence of the positive effects of TFT has been produced by a device long used in cardiological research throughout the world to measure Heart Rate Variability, or HRV. The HRV test quantifies variations in the intervals between heartbeats, which in turn are a window to the all-important autonomic nervous system (ANS).

Now, HRV has become a key to the TFT story. That's because HRV measurements have shown that Thought Field Therapy can directly influence the heart and balance the autonomic nervous system—thereby producing profound physical and psychological changes. As HRV scores improve, so do physical and psychological well-being. This finding has enormous implications for enhancing our overall health.

Charles

I first realized TFT could dramatically influence the heart while treating a patient named Charles. One morning, I received an unexpected phone call from Charles. He told me that he was calling from the intensive care unit of a distant hospital. I could hear an enormous amount of distress in his voice.

Charles didn't seem to be calling for professional advice. In fact, I sensed that perhaps he was saying good-bye.

I knew that Charles had suffered from heart problems for about six years. But apparently his situation had become much worse. For the past two days, he had been experiencing a racing heartbeat that was so fast and irregular that it had become life-threatening. His doctors had diagnosed his problem as atrial fibrillation, a condition in which the electrical signals of the heart become completely uncoordinated.

Charles had been given a number of drugs, but none of them stabilized his condition. He was now in a crisis situation. His doctors warned him that if nothing else worked by the following morning, they were going to stop his heart and then restart it with paddles—a last-ditch procedure that understandably terrified him.

I suggested that I treat Charles with Thought Field Therapy over the phone. At that time, I had never used TFT to treat atrial fibrillations. But I felt that Charles's anxiety levels were so intense that we had nothing to lose. I also knew that because TFT is a risk-free therapy, even if it didn't stabilize his rapid heart rate, it wouldn't have a negative effect.

So, over the phone, I guided Charles through a treatment with the most sophisticated form of TFT (called Voice Technology). It took three to four minutes to complete the treatment. Just as we finished, he said that he needed to hang up so his doctors could prepare him for more tests.

"Call me back when you can," I told Charles.

About forty-five minutes later, the phone rang.

"They're gone!" Charles exclaimed. "My doctors say that the fibrillations are gone!"

I was stunned. According to Charles, his doctors were astonished, too. After everything that traditional medicine offered him had failed, TFT had brought his atrial fibrillations under control. Charles was absolutely ecstatic.

The next time I saw Charles, I asked him if I could check his heart with equipment designed to evaluate his Heart Rate Variability. Charles agreed, and I took those HRV readings both before and after administering a TFT treatment. For the HRV monitoring, he merely slipped his index finger into a Velcro wrap containing a pulse sensor, which was hooked up to the HRV machinery. In just minutes, we had the results:

- Prior to the TFT treatment, Charles's HRV indicated that his autonomic nervous system was functioning in a "high sync" mode only 33 percent of the time. It was never in the "ideal zone."

- Immediately after the treatment, his "high sync" rating had soared to 79 percent. He was in the "ideal zone" *100 percent of the time*.

Charles's improvement, although dramatic, is not unusual. The thousands of people helped by Thought Field Therapy every year include an increasing number who have sought help for physical problems (in at least seven other cases, irregular heartbeats have been successfully stabilized with TFT). While TFT was initially developed for patients with psychological problems, its success in treating Charles's irregular heartbeat demonstrated that TFT also has significant physiological effects as well. If you had asked me early in TFT's development whether my algorithms for emotional distress might also heal a medical condition, I would have replied, "Probably not." But all of that has changed, thanks to HRV entering the TFT picture.

What HRV Tells Us

Although you probably aren't conscious of it, your heart functions with subtle but desirable variations between beats. We now know that measurements of this Heart Rate Variability can provide important information about your health and well-being, including the functioning of the autonomic nervous system (ANS). In fact, HRV appears to be the most accurate tool we have for monitoring the ANS, which is the internal system that controls heartbeat, breathing, body temperature, blood pressure, blood chemistry, tissue repair, metabolism, immune function, and other processes considered "involuntary" and beyond conscious control. Clearly, the more optimally your ANS is functioning, the healthier you are likely to be.

Now, with HRV technology, we can quantify the autonomic nervous system underpinnings of many physical and psychological disorders. While HRV began as a tool for cardiologists, its applications have expanded into many other medical specialties, and now into clinical psychology and psychiatry as well. It can detect subtle but often significant health-related changes at the most fundamental level. No wonder HRV has been called a window to an individual's overall health.

The HRV machine measures variations in the heart rate—not the heart rate itself, but rather the *intervals* between heartbeats—which is information needed to evaluate the workings of the autonomic nervous system. Physicians once believed (and some still do) that the rhythms of the healthy heart should be perfectly even—70 beats per minute, for example, minute after minute after minute. However, researchers have now learned that there should be variations in the heart rate, even though they may be so subtle that special technology is needed to detect them. Cardiological research has determined that the greater the variability in the heart rate, the healthier the heart and the more stable and healthy the body.

For example, let's say that two people have average heart rates of 70 beats per minute. One of them has consecutive pulse rates of 71, 68, 72, 68, 69, and 71 beats per minute—small variations from one minute to the next, and an average of 70 beats. The second individual has more pronounced variations in her heart rate—65, 75, 67, 73, 62, and 78—but still an average of 70 beats per minute. The first person, whose heart rate is more even, is said to have a more "depressed" HRV, and thus a heart status that could be more worrisome. An even interval is a danger sign and even a predictor of mortality; it is much more desirable to have a form of "chaos" taking place when it comes to those intervals.

How does Thought Field Therapy fit into this picture? In the context of TFT, Heart Rate Variability is, first and foremost, a way to monitor the effects of TFT—to evaluate what's going on in the body before and after a treatment. TFT works with or without the presence of HRV equipment to keep track of how a particular patient is doing, but the HRV has given us concrete, irrefutable evidence that TFT is producing measurable *physiological* changes even as it produces *psychological* healing. I often use HRV to evaluate TFT whether I'm trying to heal a patient's anger, grief, anxiety, or phobia, or relieve his or her physical problems such as migraine pain or allergies. HRV is an adjunct to TFT that objectively demonstrates and quantifies the effectiveness of this breakthrough therapeutic technique.

Before I had ever heard about HRV, my own background and interest in biology convinced me that Thought Field Therapy was causing deep and profound biochemical and neurological effects. But now we have a way of measuring these changes. If you have any doubts that Thought Field Therapy really can activate the body's own healing system through its simple tapping algorithms, you need only look at the measurements taken by HRV equipment before and after TFT treatments. In fact, experts in Heart Rate Variability have told me that TFT causes changes in the body more effectively than most other approaches—better than biofeedback and even many medications—and *no* treatment approach is better at rebalancing the autonomic nervous system. This viewpoint is supported by clinical research.

The Insights of Fuller Royal

While TFT's origins date back about two decades, HRV has even a longer history. It became available about thirty years ago and has been used primarily in hospitals and research centers for monitoring the well-being of the heart and the autonomic nervous system.

My own introduction to HRV came in the late 1990s, in a phone call from Fuller Royal, M.D., the respected medical director of The Nevada Clinic. Dr. Royal has turned the focus of his medical practice to alternative forms of treatment and is now president of the Nevada Board of Homeopathic Medical Examiners. In that phone call, he explained that he had been experimenting with a simple Thought Field Therapy algorithm with some of his patients, and they had achieved remarkable results in both symptomatic relief and improvements in HRV readings. No matter what each patient's particular medical condition was, Dr. Royal administered my phobia algorithm—it was the only one he knew!

Dr. Royal had heard about TFT while visiting a college in Southern California where he was lecturing. After his speech, a student asked him if he was familiar with Thought Field Therapy, which he wasn't. But, intrigued by what he was told about TFT, he obtained some TFT materials and began using the phobia algorithm with his patients.

Dr. Royal told me he had done some HRV testing before and after each TFT treatment, "and I can tell you that the effect on the autonomic nervous system is nothing short of phenomenal." He was particularly impressed with the improvements produced by TFT. "Heart Rate Variability is the only test known that will not respond to a placebo effect," he said. "You can't fool the autonomic nervous system." So, added Dr. Royal, these TFT-produced changes in HRV are *real.*

About a week later, I spent time with Dr. Royal at his clinic and observed him as he treated twelve patients with Thought Field Therapy. These people had physical problems ranging from severe pain (in a woman in her sixties) to seizure disorders (in a seven-year-old girl). In case after case, their medical condition improved. As it did, so did their HRV readings (a clear sign of autonomic nervous system changes indicative of healing).

"TFT has been for me a nice piece of the puzzle that has been missing on how to enter, and correct rapidly, defects in the autonomic nervous system," Dr. Royal says. He also believes that HRV will eventually replace many of the standard tests presently used by physicians.

The Research

Perhaps the most startling finding from the research into Heart Rate Variability is that it is a powerful indicator, and is even predictive, of an individual's *overall* health. Thus, it is a clear view not only of the present, but also of your future, well-being.

Here are capsule reviews of some of the most impressive studies of the importance of HRV to your health:

• At Washington University School of Medicine, researchers found that when HRV readings are depressed, they are an independent risk factor for death in people with heart disease. Other risk factors are more widely known, of course, and include high blood pressure, cigarette smoking, elevated blood cholesterol levels, and obesity, among others. But this study found that a low HRV score leaves you more susceptible to death.

• In the famed Framingham Heart Study, researchers have monitored the overall health status of residents of Framingham, Massachusetts, for five decades, evaluating many aspects of their well-being (not just their cardiac health). They have found that in the population at large, a depressed HRV reading is associated with a greater chance of a future heart attack, angina (chest pain), congestive heart failure, and sudden death. A large number of people in Framingham have died suddenly and unexpectedly, without knowing that they were at risk. HRV has turned out to be a stronger predictor of their death than any other indicator.

• At Harvard Medical School, a study examined the role of HRV in the well-being of nearly six hundred men suffering from anxiety. The researchers concluded that anxiety causes an alteration in the autonomic control of the heart, as well as a depressed HRV, which increases the risk of arrhythmias (irregular heartbeats) and sudden cardiac death.

• The journal *Psychiatry Research* published a study conducted at Wright State University, which evaluated patients with panic disorders. These people suffered from symptoms commonly associated with this condition, such as a pounding heart, irregular heartbeats, shortness of breath, and chest pain. When these individuals were monitored with HRV equipment, researchers found that their disorder produced low HRV readings and dysfunctions of the autonomic nervous system.

- In the Netherlands, researchers kept track of the health of 878 middle-aged men (ages forty to sixty years old). Their Heart Rate Variability was monitored periodically for twenty-five years. The investigators concluded that in the men with depressed HRV readings, their overall risk of mortality from *all* causes was higher than in men with normal HRV status. Death from noncoronary diseases, particularly cancer, contributed significantly to this increased risk.

- At Free University Hospital in Amsterdam, researchers studied twenty patients with a common form of multiple sclerosis called active-relapsing MS. These individuals were evaluated regularly with autonomic function tests consisting of HRV monitoring, as well as imaging studies (MRI) of the brain, to document the ongoing status of the disease. They found that these MS patients showed a progression of ANS dysfunction and concluded that even in the absence of changes in MRIs and in clinical symptoms, Heart Rate Variability could be a useful way to measure changes in the course of the disease.

What relevance do these studies have to Thought Field Therapy? Remember, by using a TFT algorithm like those in this book, HRV patterns can be returned to normal. When that happens, the health and well-being of the individual clearly improves.

Consider this fact: more than five hundred thousand Americans die each year from sudden cardiac death, caused primarily by fibrillations. Not all fibrillations are life-threatening (but many are), and with HRV, we have learned that Thought Field Therapy may be able to normalize the functioning of the autonomic nervous system and the heart, stabilize those high-risk fibrillations, and thus in turn perhaps significantly lower this staggering death toll.

I expect Heart Rate Variability technology to find many new applications as an adjunct to diagnosing and treating many physical and psychological disorders. For example, in 1996 a task force of the European Society of Cardiology and the North American Society of Pacing and Electrophysiology reported that changes in HRV may be an early manifestation of a number of neurological diseases, including multiple sclerosis and Parkinson's disease. In these physical conditions, periodic HRV measurements may be useful in quantifying the rate of disease progression and the effectiveness of treatments. Shifts in HRV readings may also provide clues to the course of disorders as diverse as asthma, chronic fatigue syndrome, major depression, and anorexia nervosa. Some researchers have found HRV particularly helpful in the early diagnosis of diabetic neuropathy (nerve damage associated with diabetes) and in tracking its progression; this is because neuropathy in these patients occurs in association with impairment of autonomic function.

DOCTORS AND TFT

Not long ago, I treated a fifty-nine-year-old physician named Steven. He had been diagnosed with clinical depression seven years earlier. In addition to his psychological distress, his overall physical health was poor as well. Despite long-term psychotherapy and treatment with a number of antidepressant drugs, his depression did not improve. He rated it as a 10 on the SUD (Subjective Units of Distress) scale—the highest possible level of stress. Ironically, even though he had helped thousands of patients in his own practice, no one seemed able to help him. With so many treatment failures, he had resigned himself to a life of depression and physical illness.

In 1999, Steven attended one of my training seminars, and he volunteered to be a demonstration subject. When we took an HRV reading, the results were disturbing. His total power score was 53.7. His SDNN ("standard deviation of normal-to-normal," an indicator of the variability of the heart rate) was 32.2, which was particularly worrisome (a score lower than 50 has been shown to be predictive of mortality in the near term). An HRV authority at the seminar told me that he had never seen or heard of a power score so low.

Next, I treated Steven with Thought Field Therapy, and then took another measurement with HRV. Was there a change? Yes, and a dramatic one (see chart on the following page). In just seven minutes, all traces of his depression had vanished. The second HRV showed that his power score had climbed more than a *hundred-fold*, increasing dramatically from 53.7 to 6,595.8—now well within the normal range and very close to optimum balance. At the same time, Steven's SDNN leaped from a dangerously low 32.2 to a desirable 144.4. His HRV-generated Autonomic Balance Diagram indicated that his autonomic nervous system had moved to the edges of the center square, meaning that the ANS was very close to being in balance. As these changes occurred, Steven said he subjectively felt much better; his SUD score had plummeted from a 10 to a 1 (no trace of remaining depression and hopelessness).

Not long thereafter, in an article that Steven wrote in *The Thought Field*, a newsletter devoted to TFT, he said, "I suddenly felt a bright outlook almost beyond belief. My HRV chart reflected this change. It was amazing."

Keep in mind that while these impressive improvements were reflected in the HRV printout, they were produced by Thought Field Therapy and would have occurred whether or not we had monitored the treatment with HRV. When you notice distinct, positive changes after using TFT, you would likely see corresponding improvements in Heart Rate Variability if you were hooked up to an HRV machine.

There's a postscript to this story. Early the following morning, Steven received an emergency phone call in his hotel room, and it

STEVEN'S HRV SCORES

	Before TFT	After TFT
SUD Score	10	1
SDNN on HRV	32.2	144.4
Total power on HRV	53.7	6595.8

AUTONOMIC BALANCE DIAGRAM

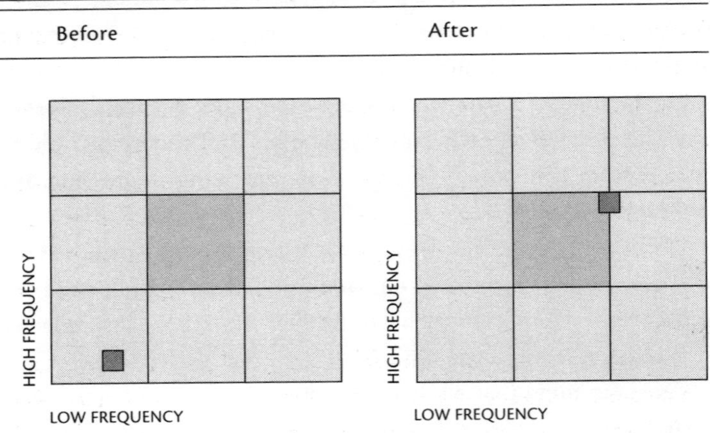

The patient is far away from autonomic balance prior to treatment. After TFT, his autonomic nervous system is much closer to balance.

brought some terrible news. His beloved daughter, Linda, had died unexpectedly. Steven and his wife, Marilyn, were in shock and immediately arranged to catch the next flight home. But while waiting for a cab to arrive for the trip to the airport, Marilyn urged him to call me from their hotel. She hoped that I might be able to ease his overwhelming grief the same way I had resolved his depression, by administering a brief TFT treatment.

When I received the call from Steven, he was fighting back tears. I told him that I understood the misery he was feeling, and although it was normal, I might be able to ease the intensity of that pain. The reality of his loss, of course, would never change. But the gut-wrenching agony surrounding Linda's death could be relieved.

In the minutes before the cab arrived, I treated Steven with TFT over the phone. It took just three minutes. As the treatment ended, his emotional distress eased.

Steven's heart was still broken and he would miss his daughter no less. But, instantly, he was more at peace with what had happened. As he said, he had "compassionate memories of my daughter instead of a devastating arrow right in the center of my heart."

Later, many of Steven's professional colleagues said they were puzzled by what had happened. They told him that to heal, he needed to "go into [his] pain," feel it intensely, and that he would need many months to feel whole again. But thanks to TFT, his emotional suffering ended almost immediately. He later wrote about his experience so others would realize what is possible.

As evidence supporting the efficacy of Thought Field Therapy accumulates, it is harder for even the most skeptical physicians and psychologists to dismiss it. With success rates unprecedented in psychotherapy, and with breakthroughs in managing physical ailments as well, a greater number of doctors are gradually approaching TFT with an open mind, wanting to know more about it, and in many cases, eager for their own patients to try it.

Anything new raises the inevitable quizzical expressions from the traditionalists. Cynicism greeted behavioral therapy, Gestalt therapy, and other new psychotherapeutic approaches at a time when psychoanalysis was the only accepted treatment. Mainstream psychotherapists, defending the status quo, argued vehemently that if you weren't doing psychoanalysis, you weren't doing *real* therapy. But despite such doubts, I personally train hundreds of health-care professionals in Thought Field Therapy each year and see their enthusiasm soar as they experience the strength of this technique and its reproducible results. Thousands of psychotherapists and other health-care professionals are now trained in TFT.

Of course, even as the evidence supporting TFT accumulates, many skeptics still exist. Some of them have argued that TFT works because of the placebo effect—that is, it is effective only because patients believe that it will work (even though HRV is reported to be free of placebo effects). But I don't hear those kinds of comments very much anymore.

I recall an incident years ago that took place in one of my own training sessions. I chose the two most skeptical psychotherapists in the group for a demonstration. One acted as the therapist, and the other volunteered to have his own severe phobia treated. The TFT algorithm was administered, and within minutes it worked. It predictably reduced the intensity of the volunteer's phobia until it had been completely eradicated. Surprised? So were the two therapists! They had to concede that their negative belief systems had no influence on TFT's effectiveness. The placebo effect certainly wasn't at play here, and in fact TFT's power overcame the militant resistance of both participants in this exercise.

Whenever a revolutionary discovery is made in science, there are strong forces at work to deny the facts, or at least approach them cautiously. It is the nature of science to be conservative. But I feel strongly that it is just as unethical to minimize a finding as it is to exaggerate it. One must be accurate. When it comes to

TFT, many more of my colleagues are now agreeing with me and are willing to take a stand that TFT has become a powerful therapeutic tool in their own practices. Remember, thousands of practitioners worldwide are now using TFT, and their patients are the ultimate beneficiaries. Using the self-help TFT algorithms in the following chapters, you'll be able to reap the healing benefits, too.

TAPPING INTO HEALING

Shortly after I was introduced to HRV, I read some research that seemed to show that making changes—particularly rapid changes—in HRV readings is virtually impossible. Two studies (one of humans, the other an animal study) found that exercise was the only common way to get those HRV scores to budge in a positive direction, but even then, it would take eight weeks or more of intense physical activity to produce improvements in SDNN scores of up to 69 percent. But then along came Thought Field Therapy. Use of the TFT algorithms in this book can cause more dramatic and more rapid positive changes in HRV readings than *any* other approach. And by doing so, they can produce physiological and psychological changes that may literally be lifesaving.

At a 1999 conference, a Norwegian authority on Heart Rate Variability reported that he was astonished at Thought Field Therapy's ability to rapidly improve HRV scores. He had tested more than ten thousand patients with HRV over the years, so he was thoroughly familiar with HRV readings—and how difficult it is to change them. But then he described the first time he evaluated TFT's effect on HRV scores. He said he was so surprised by the dramatic improvements in HRV that occurred within minutes that he believed there had been a mistake in the data he obtained; he thought perhaps his equipment was faulty. So he checked his equipment and repeated the tests. The findings were the same. Finally, he had to acknowledge the effectiveness of TFT.

This kind of initial skepticism occurs all the time. When an HRV research project was launched recently at Baylor University, the director of the program there observed a patient with arrhythmias performing a TFT algorithm. At the end of the treatment, the patient's irregular heartbeats were gone. What was the researcher's reaction? "This blows my mind!" she said. "How did you do that?"

TFT clearly produces healing in the body. Here's still another example:

On a trip to Japan in 1999, I met with a brilliant young physician who was very ill; he had been diagnosed with a serious heart condition several years ago. A month before our meeting, his heart had stopped completely for a prolonged period; fortunately, he was close to a hospital at the time, and doctors were able to start his heart again. Two months later, when I measured his HRV, his "variability" and "power" scores were alarmingly low. But then I treated him with a single TFT session. Immediately, his HRV readings returned to normal. His SDNN soared from a risky 16 up to 91. His "total power," which was initially quite low at 131, climbed to 3,019, and his autonomic nervous system was in almost perfect balance as shown in the Autonomic Balance Diagram (see charts on page 68).

Interestingly, this physician was an authority on HRV. He was stunned by his own dramatic improvements, which TFT had produced almost instantaneously.

I've seen the same kinds of positive changes occurring with TFT when the goal has been to manage stress. The hassles and headaches of everyday life can create the kind of chronic stress that undermines your physical and mental well-being. Stress speeds up and disrupts the entire physiological system, most notably shifting the sympathetic portion of your autonomic nervous system into overdrive and inundating the bloodstream with stress hormones that cause dramatic changes in the body—such as accelerating breathing and pulse rate, and increasing blood pressure.

When this so-called “fight-or-flight” response persists day after day, week after week, and even year after year, it can take a staggering toll on your well-being. As I’ve suggested, chronic stress can contribute to fatigue, insomnia, low libido, a weakened immune response, and serious health risks such as depression, heart disease, and perhaps even cancer. But Thought Field Therapy can help enormously. HRV readings have shown that treatment with TFT normalizes and balances the sympathetic and parasympathetic branches of the autonomic nervous system. As that happens, it eliminates the stress response almost immediately.

Peter Julian, a Colorado psychoneuroimmunologist and clinical director at the Mountain Wellness Group and Advanced Cardio-Logix, has used Thought Field Therapy to produce changes in HRV readings. “I haven’t seen any other treatment modality change HRV as rapidly in anxiety and depression states as TFT,” he has said. “There were very profound changes in a very short period of time (minutes). I recently saw Dr. Callahan treat a severe case of depression, and the change in the HRV within about ten minutes is the most phenomenal result in HRV that I have ever seen.”

HRV is only an instrument. But as we’ve discovered, it is an exciting one because of what we are learning about Thought Field Therapy from it. When TFT treatments are monitored with HRV, we have objective evidence that unprecedented changes have occurred in the autonomic nervous system. HRV machinery has recently become available at modest prices for home use. Remember, however, that TFT is effective whether or not you decide to monitor your progress with HRV.

I believe you’ll be hearing a lot more about Heart Rate Variability. In fact, as the power of HRV becomes more widely known, no psychotherapy will be considered valid unless its efficacy can be proven by the HRV test.

I find it thrilling that TFT has been able to produce significant *physiological* changes—confirmed by HRV—in people with serious and sometimes life-threatening conditions. TFT clearly benefits not only emotional problems but physical ones as well.

ONE PHYSICIAN'S HRV SCORES

	Before TFT	After TFT
SUD Score	10	1
SDNN on HRV	16.3	91.4
Total power on HRV	131.1	3018.7

AUTONOMIC BALANCE DIAGRAM

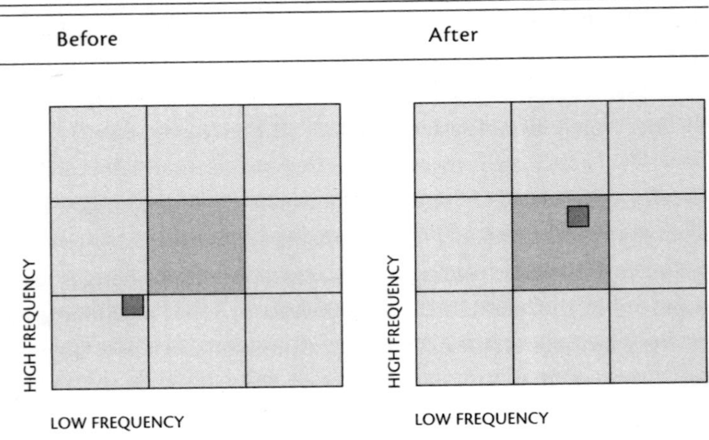

The autonomic nervous system is far out of balance prior to treatment. TFT put the autonomic system into good balance.

part two

TAPPING THE HEALER WITHIN

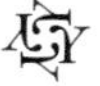

4

THE ABC'S OF ALGORITHMS

IN THIS CHAPTER, you'll become acquainted with the components of the Thought Field Therapy algorithms that you'll be using to manage your own emotional problems.

Algorithm is a term and a concept rooted in mathematics. In the context of math, it refers to a common solution to a problem (for example, a solution for finding the highest common divisor). One authority defines the more general notion of an algorithm this way: "A sequence of instructions to be followed with the intention of finding a solution to a problem. Each step must specify what steps are to be taken, and although there may be many alternate routes through the algorithm, there is only one start point and one end point."

In medicine, algorithms are treatment formulas or guidelines to be followed for diagnosing and/or managing specific diseases. They are sets of proven steps that, when followed diligently by doctors, can produce more accurate diagnoses and more efficient and successful patient care.

In TFT, algorithms are used for treatment. I developed them over time, using the Causal Diagnosis procedure unique to TFT. While it's not necessary to understand this complex process, keep in mind that each component of every algorithm was tested on hundreds of clients and shown to have a very high success rate before becoming part of this program. Only when the common efficacy of the treatment sequences could be shown did I grant them algorithm status. All of the algorithms in this book have a proven rate of success of 75 to 80 percent, and they are a way to enter the healing world of TFT with extraordinary ease.

Over the years, I developed a particular treatment pattern that works best for a given disorder. As a result, this book provides a different "recipe" for each psychological problem. For example, the precise elements and their sequence in the formula used for the fear of flying differ from those in the formula used for coping with a traumatic event like sexual abuse. If you follow the simple instructions of each algorithm (in Chapter 5), you can ease a variety of problems whenever necessary.

TFT as a whole has a unique architecture, so while the algorithms may differ in their specifics, they have common elements. In this chapter, we'll look at the components you'll see in the algorithms that you eventually try. The following sections are meant as an introduction to and explanation of these common elements; *do not actually try them out or practice them until you get to Chapter 5.* At that time, you'll learn the precise sequence of steps created for your particular problem. These next few pages should *not* be used as a "trial run," but rather as an orientation to what you'll be doing in the following chapter.

TUNING IS KEY

Every algorithm begins the same way. The first step is to intentionally think about or concentrate on the Thought Field associated with your emotional distress or problem. In essence, you'll be bringing thoughts associated with the problem into your awareness. You'll be asked to consciously think about your own particular fear, anxiety, or trauma.

Again, in other therapies it really doesn't matter what you're thinking about while you're being treated. But with TFT, it makes all the difference in the world. To be treated successfully, you need to tune the perturbed Thought Field—in other words, think about the problem that you're trying to resolve. This will bring to the fore the specific perturbations and related information that are active in the problem and need to be addressed in the treatment. In the early years of TFT, I compared this process to tuning a specific radio station. If you turn the dial to another station instead, you will get completely different information. Or imagine asking your tailor to alter your trousers without bringing the trousers to him; the job just wouldn't get done.

Psychologists have known for many years that particular thoughts have definite and profound effects on an individual. This concept is fundamental to clinical psychology. As you turn your attention to the event, circumstance, or person that is the focus of your psychological problem, it's understandable that you'll have an emotional reaction to those thoughts. But even though the process of tuning a Thought Field may make you feel distressed and upset, it's an important element in healing.

Several years ago, I appeared on a national television show called "Evening Magazine," in which I treated a woman with phobias; she had been unable to drive on freeways or over bridges for eighteen years. During that program, in a segment taped in her living room, I asked this woman to turn her attention to her driving difficulties. As she did, you could see her easygoing and relaxed demeanor change immediately to a state of high anxiety. One minute, she was having a comfortable conversation, the next, she became quite upset at the mere thought of driving across a bridge. That's the effect that tuning a Thought Field can have. (By the way, after a brief TFT treatment, her phobia was gone without a trace, and she no longer felt *any* anxiety when thinking about her former fears. In fact, with the cameras rolling, she got into her car and drove on a freeway and over two bridges, calmly and without a bit of fear.)

In the next chapter, when you tune a Thought Field and it produces intense emotions, this will be a clear indication that perturbations exist. These perturbations will appear immediately upon tuning the Thought Field. When I was developing TFT, I would give patients plenty of time to tune the Thought Field. I'd watch their eyes and their facial expression to make sure they really had it. I later learned that the tuning takes place instantly. If you don't become upset, there are probably no perturbations present, although there are exceptions. Most notably, a person repressing his psychological problem may not become distressed merely thinking about it; however, if he were to be exposed to the actual situation—for example, speaking in public—then his anxiety would surface. (The Causal Diagnosis procedure of TFT can identify precisely what perturbations are present, allowing even a repressed person to be treated successfully.)

RATING THE DISTRESS LEVEL

Once you've tuned the Thought Field, you'll be asked to rate your psychological turmoil on the Subjective Units of Distress (SUD) scale. The SUD, as you'll recall, is a widely accepted psychological tool. It is a simple 10-point scale, with 10 being the worst you could possibly feel, and 1 indicating absolutely no trace of upset. The SUD can be used for any kind of human problem as a way of quantifying the intensity of your feelings, emotions, stress, or pain.

The SUD will give you some valuable information as you begin the self-treatment process, with no confusion about where you stand. Perhaps you recall the scene in the movie *Annie Hall*, in which the characters played by Woody Allen and Diane Keaton are shown on a split screen while each is responding to a question from their respective psychotherapists about their sex lives. Keaton's answer is, "It's terrible; we have sex all the time!" How frequently? "Twice a week," she says. Allen responds to the same questions: "We never have sex!" How infrequently? "Twice a week." This scene shows how two people can perceive and describe the same life experience very differently. In TFT, it's valuable to have a numerical scale that sidesteps the problems that can occur in interpreting the meanings of words. Psychologists have created a number of elaborate scales and inventories to assess how a particular patient is doing. But frankly, most are just very complicated ways of asking the same question that you'll be answering with the SUD scale: "How are you feeling?"

So as part of each TFT algorithm in Chapter 5, you'll be asked to quantify the intensity of your upset or discomfort. While thinking about the emotional problem in your life, you'll rate the degree of your distress *at that moment* on the 10-point scale and then *write it down*. Unless you commit it to paper, you'll be surprised how easy it is to forget after the treatment how intense your pain was. I believe that there is no adequate substitute for this kind of personal assessment. *You* are the expert on how you feel. So be as honest and accurate as you can when evaluating your emotions and assigning a numerical value to them.

You'll be asked to take SUD ratings two or more times—during the algorithm itself, and again at its completion to assess the degree of improvement that you've made. Each time you should write down the new SUD. Each SUD will provide immediate feedback on the effectiveness of the treatment and may help determine the next step in the treatment process. In some cases, the SUD value may indicate that it's time to move to the gamut series (discussed in the following pages). But if improvements seem slow or stalled, you may be experiencing what is called *psychological reversal* (PR), and you'll be asked to perform the PR correction described later in this chapter.

TAPPING

Every TFT algorithm contains a series of tapping maneuvers on carefully chosen points on the body. The initial points in the algorithm are considered the *majors* of TFT. The tapping actually stimulates changes in the body's energy flow that can influence the particular problem being treated through an effect on the perturbations (the fundamental cause of the problem).

FIGURE 4.1

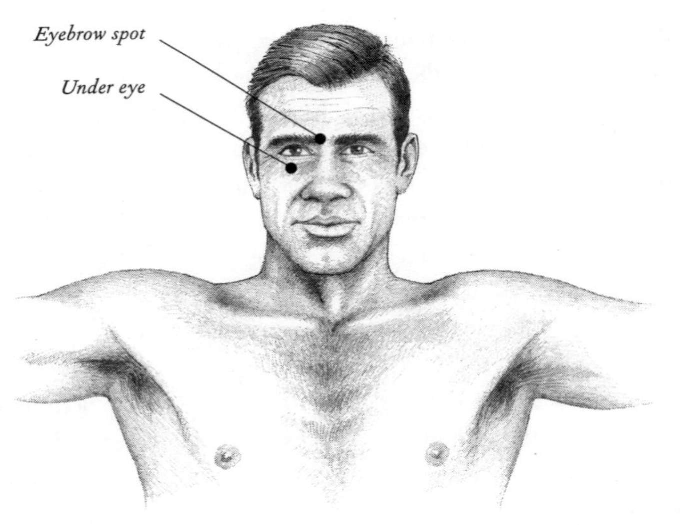

In Chapter 5, depending on your specific emotional distress, you might be instructed to do several of the following steps with your problem in mind:

- Use two fingers of one hand (either hand is OK) to tap a spot at the beginning of the eyebrow, just above the bridge of the nose. Tap five times, firmly and gently, not nearly hard enough for it to hurt or bruise, but solidly enough to stimulate the energy flow in the system. (See Figure 4.1.)
- Tap five times under the eye, about an inch below the bottom of the eyeball, at the bottom of the center of the bony orbit, high on the cheek. Tap firmly, but not hard enough to cause pain. (See Figure 4.1.)

FIGURE 4.2

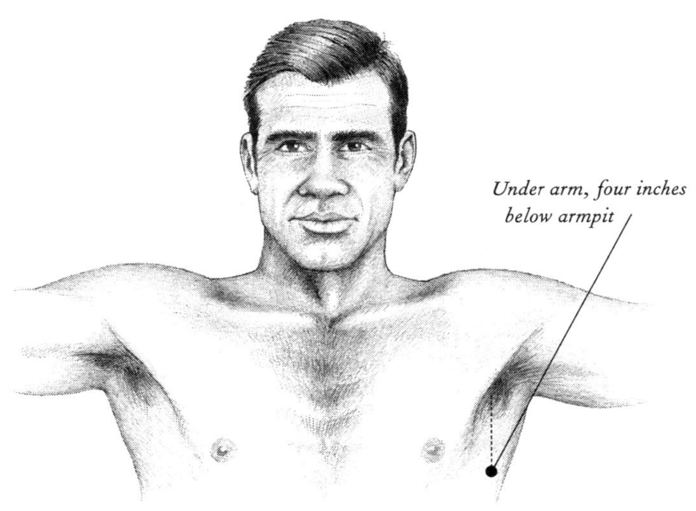

- Tap solidly several times under the arm, about four inches directly below the armpit, using rigid fingers. In men, this spot is under the arm about even with the nipple. Women can locate this spot by tapping at about the center of the bra strap under the arm. (See Figure 4.2.)
- Tap the "collarbone point." To locate it, take two fingers of either hand and run them down the center of the throat to the top of the center collarbone notch. This is approximately even with the spot where a man would knot his tie. From there, move straight down an additional inch. Then move to the right one inch. Tap this point five times. (See Figure 4.3.)
- Tap the "little finger spot." It is located on the inside tip of the finger, adjacent to the nail, and on the side of the finger next to the ring finger. Tap this point five times. (See Figure 4.4.)

FIGURE 4.3

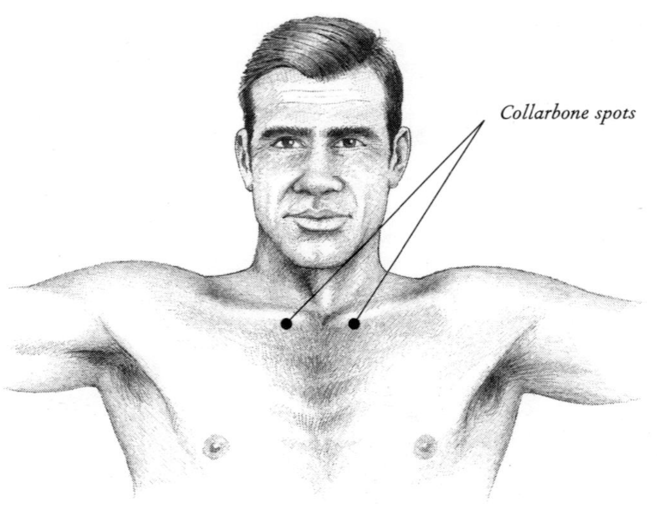

- Tap the "index finger spot." It is located on the tip of the index (pointing) finger, on the side of that finger next to the thumb. Tap this point five times. (See Figure 4.4.)

Again, don't hurt yourself with these tapping maneuvers when you actually perform them in Chapter 5. Find a tapping intensity that is firm but gentle.

The results achieved with these tapping maneuvers and TFT in general are quite predictable, and improvement tends to occur in quantum leaps. The initial tapping motions will typically produce a decline in the SUD of 2 or more points when the SUD began at 7 or greater. So, for example, a frequent decrease is from 10 to 7, or 10 to 5, or even 10 to 1. At the end of the algorithm, the SUD will have declined to 1 in most people, indicating that the upset has been completely eliminated. These declines will occur no matter how familiar or unfamiliar you were with TFT before the therapy began.

FIGURE 4.4

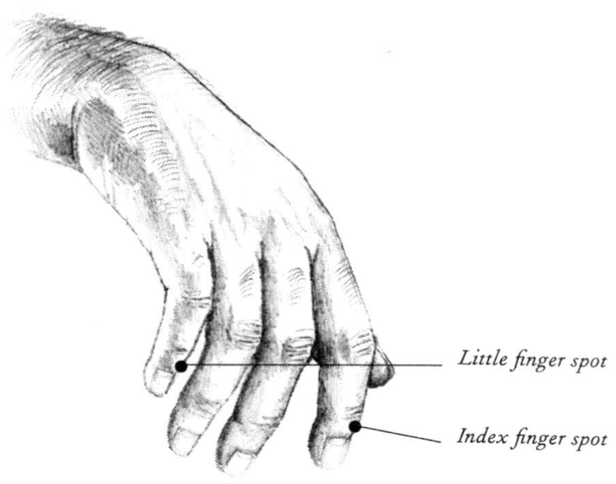

THE GAMUT SERIES

The gamut series is a group of nine rapid treatments performed while tapping the "gamut spot" on the back of the hand. To locate this point, make a fist with your nondominant hand and note the knuckles standing out on the back of the hand. Place the index finger of your dominant hand in the valley between the knuckles of the ring finger and the little finger. Now open your hand. Then move the index finger about one inch down toward the wrist. This is the gamut point. (See Figure 4.5.)

When instructed to do so in Chapter 5, you should tap the gamut point continuously with two fingers of the opposite hand, tapping firmly but gently about three to five times per second. Continue this tapping while proceeding through all nine of the gamut treatments, tapping about five to six times for each of the nine treat-

FIGURE 4.5

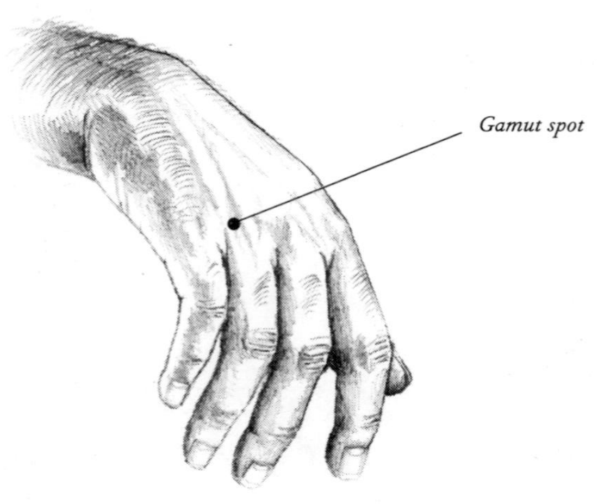

ments. Six of these treatments involve particular eye movements and eye positions. The remaining three involve humming and counting.

Why eye movements? The eye is an extension of the brain, and I believe that each eye movement may access a different area of the brain. Some research shows, for example, that when the eyes are open, the back of the brain receives relatively greater stimulation; when they are closed, the front of the brain is more stimulated. Eye movements have been used in other health-related disciplines, including neurolinguistic programming (NLP), applied kinesiology, and the Feldenkreis method. NLP practitioners, for example, claim that certain eye movements allow access to particular memories. In my own TFT research, I recognized that the position of the eyes could diagnostically reveal a hidden perturbation. I also discovered that tapping the gamut point while moving the eyes in particular ways could contribute to a collapsing of a perturbation, immediately minimizing or eradicating a psychological problem.

The humming and counting processes are designed to activate the right and left brain, respectively. Theoretically, the right side of the brain is being receptive to treatment by the humming and tapping, and the left side of the brain by the counting and tapping.

Here are the nine gamut treatments (see Figures 4.6 through 4.11):

1. Open the eyes.
2. Close the eyes.
3. Open the eyes and point them down and to the left.
4. Point the eyes down and to the right.
5. Whirl the eyes around in a circle in one direction.
6. Whirl the eyes around in the opposite direction. Rest the eyes.

FIGURES 4.6–4.11

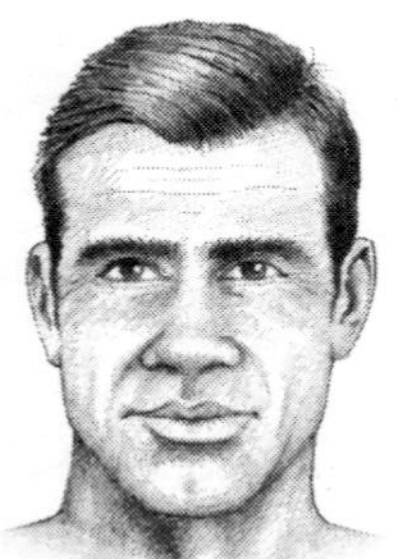

FIGURE 4.6

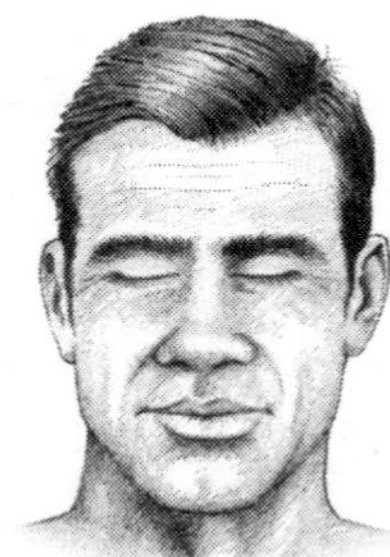

FIGURE 4.7

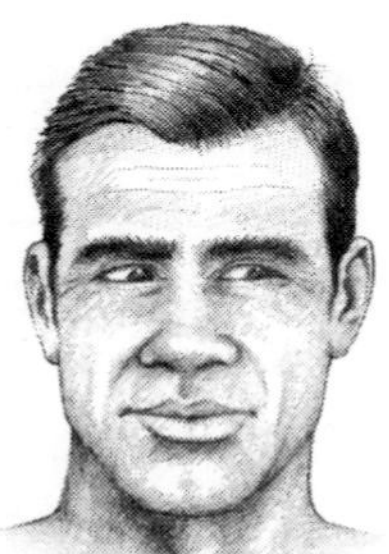

FIGURE 4.8

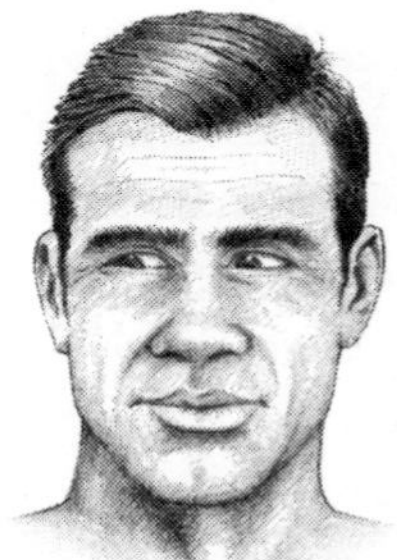

FIGURE 4.9

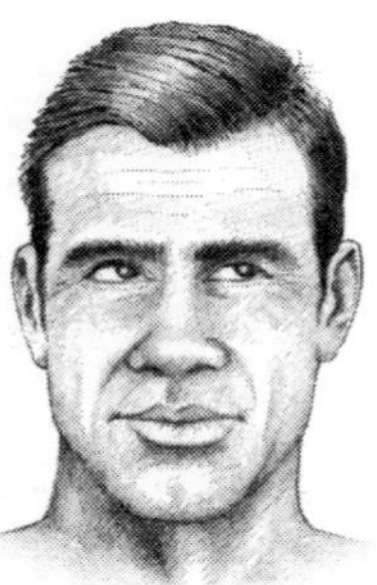

FIGURE 4.10

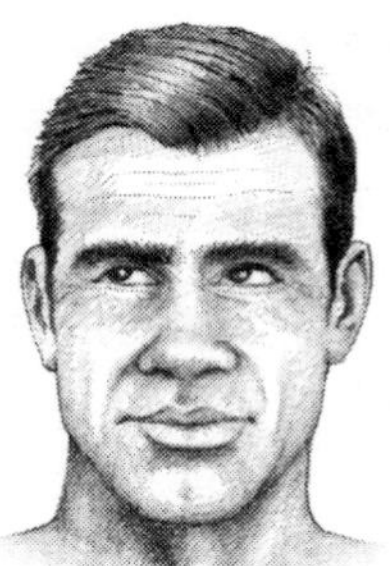

FIGURE 4.11

7. Hum a few bars of any tune aloud (more than a single note).

8. Count aloud from one to five.

9. Hum the tune again.

By the way, I selected the word *gamut* because, as you can see above, a wide range of treatments are performed while tapping this one spot (the "gamut point"). *Remember to continue tapping the gamut point while performing all nine steps.*

If you have a disability that prevents you from performing any of the eye movements—for example, if you are blind—simply imagine doing those movements while tapping the gamut spot. In the same way, if you are unable to hum and count aloud, perhaps because you are in a public place, you can imagine humming and counting.

FLOOR-TO-CEILING EYE ROLL

This step is one of my most recent discoveries. It is generally the final treatment in the TFT algorithm, performed after the earlier steps have produced their improvements in the SUD score. At this point, most individuals have reduced their SUD to a 1 or 2. The floor-to-ceiling eye roll is a way to solidify this improvement—to either strengthen the 1 rating, or reduce the 2 to a 1.

Remember, the eyes are an extension of the brain. Research has shown that when the eyes are moved according to the following instructions, most people will experience further improvement in their condition. Perform this maneuver as follows:

Hold your head level, and move your eyes down. Then begin tapping the gamut point as you move your eyes upward.

This process should take only about six to seven seconds. Remember to keep tapping the gamut spot as you move the eyes upward.

PSYCHOLOGICAL REVERSAL

If you're not getting maximum results from TFT, it could be caused by *psychological reversal*, or PR. Psychological reversal is the most common reason that healing does not take place, keeping an otherwise effective therapy from working.

What's the cause of psychological reversal? It appears that PR is associated with a reversal of polarity in the meridian system. In other words, your internal energy flow has actually become reversed or, in some cases, blocked. If you have a negative, self-critical attitude or self-sabotaging behavior, this could be a sign that PR is present.

By treating psychological reversal, you can dissolve the energy-flow disruptions that have interfered with TFT. This is not a therapy for the underlying psychological problem itself, but rather for the obstacles that are preventing the primary TFT treatment from being effective. This PR correction can work within seconds, thus contributing significantly to the chances for success with TFT.

Here's how to correct a psychological reversal:

1. Find what I call the "PR spot." It is located on the outside edge of the hand, about midway between the wrist and the base of the little finger. This is the point where you might make contact when delivering a "karate chop." (See Figure 4.12.)

2. Tap this point five times with two fingers of the opposite hand.

Once this treatment is completed, you'll be instructed to repeat the tapping motions and SUD rating. Remember, the correction for PR does not treat the original problem you're trying to resolve, but rather eliminates the barriers to that treatment. So once the reversal is resolved, the primary treatment needs to be repeated.

Mini PR

A related procedure, called a *mini psychological reversal correction*, can be used when you decrease your SUD to a 3 or 4 but can't seem to get it any lower. In other words, you've achieved substantial improvement, but you can't get to the finish line. A block exists that is keeping you from reducing the SUD any further.

In the algorithm for your particular emotional problem, you'll be instructed on whether and when to use this technique. Here is the procedure to follow:

- Find the PR spot mentioned above, located on the outside edge of the hand, between the wrist and the base of the little finger.
- Tap about fifteen times with two fingers of the opposite hand.

FIGURE 4.12

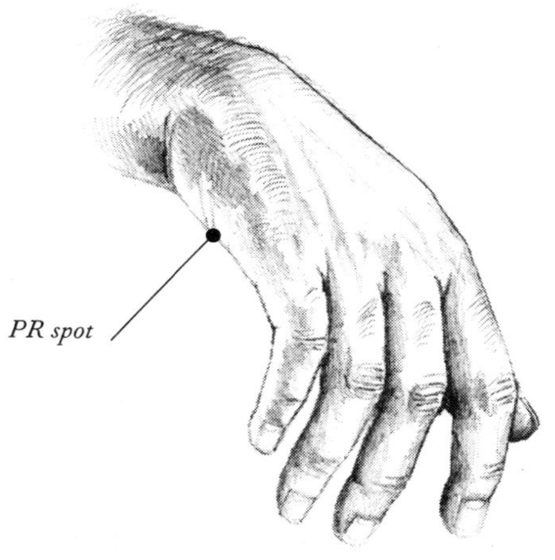

As long as a psychological reversal persists, TFT (or any other treatment) won't be able to get the SUD to a 1. The PR or mini PR correction will open the door that allows TFT to eradicate your problem.

I'll discuss other aspects of psychological reversal in more detail in Chapters 5 and 6.

THE COLLARBONE/BREATHING EXERCISE

Once you've finished using an algorithm, including the PR corrections as instructed, occasionally the SUD still may not have dropped to 1. At that point, you will have another option for eliminating your problem: the collarbone/breathing exercise. It involves five breathing positions and a series of touching and tapping maneuvers.

You'll use two "collarbone points," one of which is the same one I described earlier in the "collarbone point" tapping procedure. To locate both of the points used in this new exercise, take two fingers, one on either hand, and run them down the center of the throat to the top of the center collarbone notch. This is about where a man might knot his tie. From there, move straight down an additional inch. Then find the two TFT collarbone points, which are about one inch to the right of center and one inch to the left of center. (See Figure 4.13.) Once you have located these points, proceed with the following breathing techniques and touching and tapping procedures.

Breathing Techniques

There are five breathing positions in this exercise, to be followed in this order:

1. Breathe normally.

2. Take in a full, deep breath, and hold it.
3. Let out about half of that breath, and hold it.
4. Let out the remainder of the breath, and hold it.
5. Take in a half breath, hold it, and then release it.

THE TOUCHING STEPS

These touching steps should be performed while moving through the breathing techniques above. Start with either hand.

1. Using two fingertips, touch one of the collarbone points. As you do, tap the gamut spot of that same hand with two fingertips of the opposite hand. Simultaneously, proceed

FIGURE 4.13

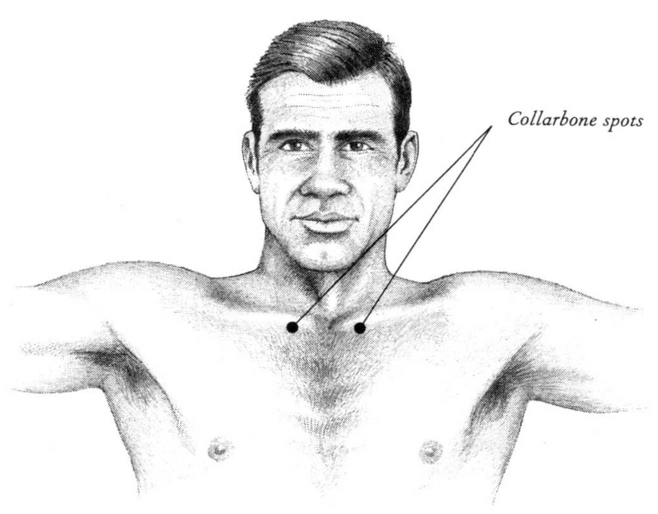

through the five breathing techniques. Tap rapidly, about five good taps for each of the five breathing steps.

2. Move the same two fingertips from the original collarbone point to the other collarbone point. Then repeat the tapping and breathing maneuvers in step 1.

3. Bend the same two "touching" fingers at the knuckle (as though you were making a fist with them), and place these knuckles so they're touching the first collarbone point. At the same time, tap the gamut spot of that hand and proceed through the five breathing techniques as described in step 1.

4. Move the same knuckles to the other collarbone point and tap the gamut spot of that hand while going through the five breathing steps.

5. Now, it's time to reverse the positions of the hands and their activity. To begin, take the fingertips of the opposite hand and touch one of the collarbone points. As you do, tap the gamut spot of that same hand with two fingertips of the other hand. Simultaneously, proceed through the five breathing techniques. Tap rapidly about five good taps for each of the five breathing steps.

6. Move the same two fingertips you began with in step 5 to touch the other collarbone point. Then repeat the tapping and breathing maneuvers as described in step 5.

7. Bend the same two "touching" fingers at the knuckle (as though you were making a fist with them), and place these knuckles so they're touching the first collarbone point. At the same time, tap the gamut spot of that hand and proceed through the five breathing steps.

8. Move the same knuckles to the other collarbone point and tap the gamut spot of that hand while going through the five breathing steps.

In all, there are forty breathing and forty tapping movements (twenty with the fingertips and twenty with the knuckles).

NORMA'S STORY

Just how successful can TFT algorithms be? Consider the case of Norma, who is typical of those whom I have treated with Thought Field Therapy. She sought my help when she was in her early forties. She could point to many successes in her life, including a thriving career as a real estate agent. She also had maintained her body weight in a healthy range of 118 to 126 pounds for many years. But then Norma went through a divorce, which changed her entire life—including her ability to control her weight. "I was living alone for the first time in my life," she said. "To make things worse, my entire family blamed me for the divorce." As if there wasn't enough new anxiety in her life, Norma smashed up her car—a Ferrari that she had absolutely cherished. The insurance company fought her on the settlement, and she ended up going to court over it.

In response to this tidal wave of stressful events, Norma began eating . . . and eating . . . and eating. Even when she wasn't hungry, she kept the refrigerator door active for hours every night. Instead of reaching for low-fat foods, she sought comfort in junk food. Her weight soared, peaking at 158 pounds.

For eight years, Norma futilely attempted to lose those excess pounds. She adopted one fad diet after another, each one ultimately failing once its novelty wore off. She also tried hypnosis. She took tranquilizers to ease her anxiety. Then she entered emotionally painful and expensive psychotherapy. Years went by, but as her frustration and her therapy bills grew, her body size remained stubbornly where it was. When she called my office, there was despair in her voice. She was at wit's end.

I told Norma about Thought Field Therapy, and she agreed to try it. In my office, I asked her to focus on her desire for junk food, and then to rate that craving on the SUD scale of 1 to 10. She placed it at an 8. Then I guided her through the tapping of carefully chosen locations on the face and upper body, followed by the other components of the treatment. The entire process took less than five minutes.

When we were done, I asked Norma, "On a 10-point scale, what's your desire to eat junk food now?"

She thought for a moment.

"One," she finally said matter-of-factly. "I don't feel the urge at all." Instantly, she felt in control.

Each time I checked back with Norma in the following days and weeks, she reported that her relationship with food had normalized. Her obsession with eating had ended. She had stopped bingeing. And she began to lose weight. "I no longer faced a mental battle to keep from eating when I wasn't hungry," Norma told me later. "I could walk away from junk food for the first time in years."

Norma lost eight pounds in the first two months after undergoing a single TFT treatment. Within six months, she had lost a total of twenty-five pounds. "At last," she said, "I've found something that works!"

Results like Norma's are very predictable if you follow my instructions carefully. Quantum-type leaps in the SUD scale happen in individual after individual. As you move from 10 to 7 to 4 to 1, all in a matter of minutes, you are experiencing the dramatic improvements that we find typical in the thousands of people helped by TFT.

During the development of TFT, the final judgment of its effectiveness was the answer to the question, "Did it lower the SUD?" A *cure* for a psychological problem would be the complete elimination of all distress, which translates to a 1 on the SUD scale. TFT has proven it can do that in one patient after another.

5

PUTTING THE ALGORITHMS TO WORK

We've reached the "hands-on" portion of the program. It's finally time to put the algorithms to work—to use the "recipes" that can produce rapid and lasting healing of your emotional distress, and even your physical discomfort. Whether you've been struggling with this problem for weeks or for most of your lifetime, these algorithms have the power to eradicate it in minutes. Like a skilled surgeon with steady hands and a fine-tuned scalpel, you can use the algorithms to excise the distress that has disrupted your life for so long.

As I explained in Chapter 4, each algorithm is composed of a series of tapping maneuvers and other steps that need to be followed carefully. The recipe for every problem is unique and has been carefully formulated and tested for that specific condition. Though many of the same tapping maneuvers appear in one algorithm after another, the selection and sequence of steps vary from one recipe to the next. The algorithm for anxiety is different from the one for anger; the algorithm for depression is different from the one for obsession.

Turn to the particular disorder you'd like to treat, and before actually using the algorithm, read through it from beginning to end. Become completely familiar with it. If you'd like, isolate each step and try it out. Tap at the edge of the eyebrow. Tap under the eye. Find the "collarbone point" and practice tapping it. Once you become comfortable with each step, you're ready to implement the entire algorithm.

To enjoy the recipe's full benefits, you need to use it exactly as it appears. Otherwise, you may weaken its power. I've worked with some clients who had heard a little about TFT and had tried tapping randomly on their own, with little or no change in their condition. The haphazard order of their tapping, and their indiscriminate choices of points to tap, did not produce the healing they sought. I once worked with a trainee in Canada who had chronic fatigue and who had been tapping TFT points—but in a random order that did not coincide with any particular algorithm. He did this experimentally for five hours—not easy to do when fatigued—to see if he could produce any changes, but he was unable to elicit even the slightest improvement. But then (through the use of Causal Diagnosis) I determined the optimal tapping sequence for his condition; in minutes, he finally got the powerful results commonly seen with TFT.

As you turn to the section that focuses on your own particular emotional (or in one case, physical) problem and begin to use the algorithm, here are some important points to keep in mind:

- At the beginning of each algorithm, you should determine the amount of distress you're feeling while "tuning," or thinking about, your problem. It is wise to write down the SUD at that point, since once they've been cured, some people forget that they even had the emotional difficulty at all. (This is due to the Apex Problem, which I'll discuss in Chapter 7.) As you'll see in these algorithms, you'll be guided toward taking another SUD reading about midway through the recipe, and then again at the end to assess how you've fared. Be sure to write down the SUD rating each time.

- For some disorders, you'll notice that there are two or more algorithms. For example, there is an algorithm for "simple anxiety" and another for "complex anxiety"; there is an algorithm for "simple trauma" and another for "complex trauma." That's because I've discovered that complex cases require a slightly different treatment pattern than simple cases. Although Causal Diagnosis—one of the advanced Thought Field Therapy techniques—can quickly determine whether your problem is simple or complex, this isn't something you can do on your own. So the best strategy for self-management of these conditions is to begin with the "simple" recipe. Many people will notice a significant and immediate improvement after its use. However, if after completing the treatment you haven't been able to reduce your SUD score to 1, then try the "complex" algorithm. The chances are very good that you'll see not only a much more significant improvement, but a lowering of the SUD all the way down to 1. (By the way, I've often defined a "complex" case as one that takes more than five minutes to cure. That's not just a whimsical remark—I've found that if an algorithm doesn't reduce your SUD to 1 in a few minutes, and you are certain that you have done the procedures accurately, almost by definition your problem is complex.)

In the same way, a few conditions—addictive urges, panic attacks, complex anxiety, and obsession—have a "first use" algorithm, and then alternative algorithms. Again, try the "first use" treatment first; if it doesn't completely resolve the problem, then move on to the alternative recipe.

- Make sure you are choosing the right algorithm. This is particularly important for conditions such as phobias and trauma.

Although you'll find an algorithm appropriate for simple phobias, there is a separate recipe for fear of spiders, claustrophobia, and turbulence. Make sure you select the applicable algorithm. And not only are there algorithms for "simple" and "complex" trauma, but a "complex trauma" can have complicating factors that require a specific algorithm. For instance, you'll find algorithms for "complex trauma with anger" and "complex trauma with guilt." Choose the algorithm that most closely describes your problem.

- When using an algorithm, if the SUD rating doesn't decrease dramatically, bear in mind that a psychological reversal (PR) may be present that needs correcting. In this case, turn back to Chapter 4 (specifically, pages 84–86) for a description of how to use the PR and mini PR correction. These corrective processes do not reduce the SUD on their own, but once the correction is made, it clears the path so the algorithm can be repeated, which should reduce the SUD to 1.

- If you've completed every step of an algorithm and you still have a SUD of 3 or greater, then you should consider using the collarbone/breathing exercise. As you'll recall, this technique involves five breathing positions, combined with a series of tapping and touching maneuvers. To refresh your memory of how to perform the collarbone/breathing exercise, see Chapter 4 (page 86).

As you prepare to work with one or more of these algorithms, look through the illustrations in Figures 5.1 and 5.2 to refresh your memory on the key elements of these recipes. Remember, the algorithms were used successfully by hundreds of people before they were formally incorporated into the TFT program. There is no guesswork involved, and thus you shouldn't "improvise" as you use them. Each algorithm makes clear what you need to do to facilitate recovery. By paying attention to and following every step, you will give yourself the optimum opportunity for healing.

FIGURE 5.1

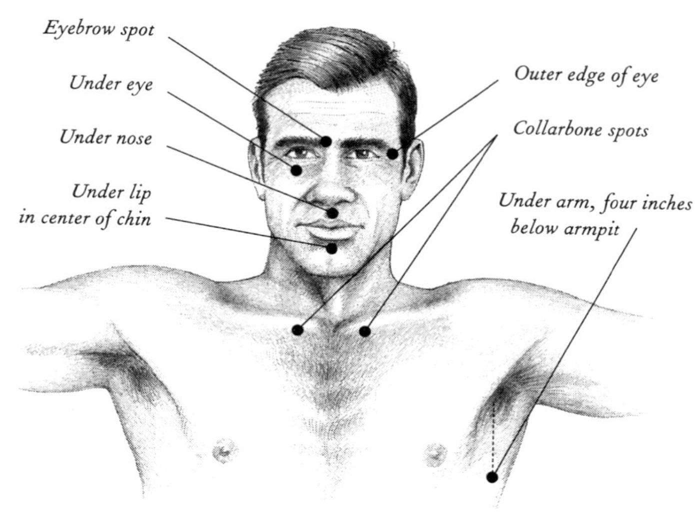

FIGURE 5.2

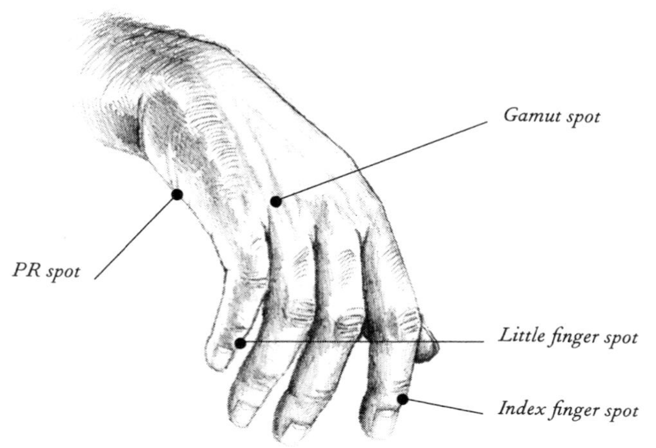

Now, in the pages that follow, find the particular problem that you want to treat and get started. Within minutes, you can experience healing that may have eluded you for years.

TRAUMA

Trauma is different from most of the other psychological problems for which I've developed algorithms. While most disorders are irrational or unrealistic (for example, people with phobias generally recognize that their fear doesn't make sense), trauma is perfectly understandable. When a traumatic event or situation occurs—such as a rape or the death of a loved one in an accident—a psychologically disturbed response is not surprising, and is even normal. Why wouldn't you be terribly upset or "traumatized" when life presents you with this kind of shock?

But the aftershocks of trauma can disrupt a life for decades. People often still become very distressed when they think about the traumatic event five, ten, and twenty years later. They may still be tormented by the departure of a spouse who left them for a new partner (so-called love pain). They may still be suffering over the death of a child.

Perhaps you've heard the story about the young woman who arrives at work in the morning and is welcomed by a male coworker with a good-natured "Good morning." Upon hearing the friendly greeting, however, she begins to cry uncontrollably. It seems that she had broken up with her boyfriend not long ago—a very traumatic event in her life. Amid the tears, she sobs, "*He* used to say that to me!"

No matter what the trauma, TFT can quiet the storm and allow you to go on with your life in a positive way.

Even the most difficult cases can be resolved with TFT. I recall treating an eight-year-old girl named Marcia who had been victimized five years earlier with severe sexual and ritualistic abuse at her preschool. The trauma was compounded in her own home, where she was abused by a man with whom her mother had been living. When I saw Marcia, she had already been in traditional psychotherapy for five years (since the age of three), but had shown no real improvement. The traumas in her past were still so upsetting that she had never been able to talk openly to anyone about them, including her mother and the series of therapists she had seen. Whenever the subject was raised, she was traumatized all over again. In fact, the nightmares that had begun years earlier seemed only to worsen over time. She had become terrified of strangers, developed a fear of dark places, and couldn't go to the bathroom or into certain rooms of her own home alone.

Although Marcia's mother was referred to me by a friend, she was initially very skeptical of TFT. But then I was able to help her rapidly eliminate her own fear of public speaking. That broke down her resistance to having me work with her daughter. She was particularly comforted by the fact that, unlike traditional therapy, TFT does not require an individual to talk about and relive difficult experiences.

I had two sessions with Marcia. We began by eradicating the fears she had developed over the years. Then we eliminated the perturbations related to the sexual abuse itself. When we were done, Marcia was visibly much more relaxed. In the ensuing weeks and months, her mother told me that Marcia had become comfortable around people and was no longer afraid to go into certain parts of their home. When I last spoke with her mother, two years later, Marcia was still doing very well.

Remember, the following TFT algorithms will not extinguish the memories of the trauma you've experienced. You'll still remember everything that happened. But they will collapse the perturbations that were seared into the Thought Field during the terrible event and that are responsible for the symptoms that have disrupted your life for so long. The memories won't have the emotional power they once did.

If you're experiencing "love pain," the algorithm for trauma should help. Throughout my years of practicing psychotherapy, I've found that even though romantic disappointments may not be the most objectively traumatic event in people's lives, they *do* cause the most devastating emotional pain. When romantic love turns sour, we typically spend weeks, months, and even years nursing our crushed hearts and spirits. We play and replay what we did and what we could have done differently to keep the love intact and prevent the breakup ("If only I'd been more affectionate . . ."; "If only I'd shown more interest in what he was interested in . . .").

The grim reality is that when a romantic relationship dies, it is thoroughly appropriate for you to be terribly upset and experience shock waves in its wake. But it is also important for you to eliminate the pain that is making it so difficult to get on with your day-to-day life. Now, TFT can eradicate *all* traces of that emotional turmoil associated with troubled relationships—and do it in minutes.

In the following pages, I've provided four algorithms for trauma. The first will work for most people and is designed for "simple trauma." Start with this algorithm. It should collapse your perturbations and reduce the SUD to 1. If it doesn't, however, then move on to the most appropriate of three algorithms for "complex trauma": complex trauma, complex trauma with anger, or complex trauma with guilt.

Simple Trauma Algorithm

1. Tune the Thought Field—that is, intentionally think about the traumatic event that produces such emotional distress in your life.

2. Rate your distress level at this moment, using the Subjective Units of Distress (SUD) scale. On this scale, 10 is the worst you could possibly feel, and 1 indicates absolutely no trace of upset. Write down the SUD rating.

3. Using two fingers of one hand, tap a spot at the beginning of the eyebrow, just above the bridge of the nose. Tap five times, firmly and gently, not nearly hard enough to bruise, but solidly enough to stimulate the energy flow in the system.

4. Tap the "collarbone point." To locate it, take two fingers of either hand and run them down the center of the throat to the top of the center collarbone notch. This is approximately even with the spot where a man would knot his tie. From there, move straight down an additional inch. Then move to the right one inch. Tap this point five times.

5. Take a second SUD rating and write it down. If the SUD has decreased 2 or more points (which will be the case for most people), then continue with step 6 below. If there was no change, however, or if the change in the SUD was only 1 point, perform the correction for a psychological reversal, using the technique described in Chapter 4 (see page 84). Then repeat steps 1 through 5.

6. Perform the nine gamut treatments. Locate the gamut spot on the back of the hand, about an inch below the raised knuckles of the ring finger and little finger when making a fist. Begin tapping the gamut spot with two fingers of the opposite hand, about three to five times per second, and continue tapping while performing all nine steps below (tap five or six times for each of the nine gamut positions). *It is very important to tap the gamut spot throughout all nine of these gamut treatments*:

   - Open the eyes.
   - Close the eyes.
   - Open the eyes and point them down and to the left.
   - Point the eyes down and to the right.

- Whirl the eyes around in a circle in one direction.
- Whirl the eyes around in the opposite direction.
- Hum a few bars of any tune aloud (more than a single note; rest the eyes).
- Count aloud from one to five.
- Hum the tune again.

7. Tap the spot at the beginning of the eyebrow again. Tap five times, firmly and gently.
8. Tap the collarbone point five times again.
9. Take still another SUD rating and write it down. If it has declined to 1 (which will happen with most people), move to step 10 below. But if it has decreased significantly yet is still not a 1, perform the mini PR correction as described in Chapter 4 (see page 85), and then repeat the treatment steps above.
10. To ensure that the improvements you've made are complete, perform the floor-to-ceiling eye roll (when the SUD is 2 or lower): Hold the head level and move your eyes down. Then begin tapping the gamut point as you move your eyes upward.

Complex Trauma Algorithm

1. Tune the Thought Field—that is, intentionally think about the traumatic event that produces such emotional distress in your life.
2. Rate your distress level at this moment, using the Subjective Units of Distress (SUD) scale. On this scale, 10

is the worst you could possibly feel, and 1 indicates absolutely no trace of upset. Write down the SUD rating.

3. Using two fingers of one hand, tap a spot at the beginning of the eyebrow, just above the bridge of the nose. Tap five times, firmly and gently, not nearly hard enough to bruise, but solidly enough to stimulate the energy flow in the system.

4. Tap five times under the eye, about an inch below the bottom of the eyeball, at the bottom of the center of the bony orbit, high on the cheek. Tap firmly, but not hard enough to cause pain.

5. Tap solidly five times under the arm, about four inches directly below the armpit, using rigid fingers. In men, this spot is under the arm about even with the nipple. Women can locate this spot by tapping at about the center of the bra under the arm.

6. Tap the "collarbone point." To locate it, take two fingers of either hand and run them down the center of the throat to the top of the center collarbone notch. This is approximately even with the spot where a man would knot his tie. From there, move straight down an additional inch. Then move to the right one inch. Tap this point five times.

7. Take a second SUD rating and write it down. If it has decreased 2 or more points (which will be the case for most people), then continue with step 8 below. If there was no change, however, or if the change in the SUD was only 1 point, perform the correction for a psychological reversal, using the technique described in Chapter 4 (see page 84). Then repeat steps 1 through 7.

8. Perform the nine gamut treatments. Locate the gamut spot on the back of the hand, about an inch below the raised knuckles of the ring finger and little finger when making a fist. Begin tapping the gamut spot with two fingers of the opposite hand, about three to five times per second, and continue tapping while performing all nine steps below (tap five or six times for each of the nine gamut positions). It is very important to tap the gamut spot throughout all nine of these gamut treatments:

   - Open the eyes.
   - Close the eyes.
   - Open the eyes and point them down and to the left.
   - Point the eyes down and to the right.
   - Whirl the eyes around in a circle in one direction.
   - Whirl the eyes around in the opposite direction.
   - Hum a few bars of any tune aloud (more than a single note; rest the eyes).
   - Count aloud from one to five.
   - Hum the tune again.

9. Tap the spot at the beginning of the eyebrow again. Tap five times, firmly and gently.
10. Tap under the eye five times again.
11. Tap solidly five times under the arm again.
12. Tap the collarbone point five times again.
13. Take still another SUD rating and write it down. If it has declined to 1 (which will happen with most people), move

to step 14 below. But if it has decreased significantly yet is still not a 1, perform the mini PR correction as described in Chapter 4 (see page 85), and then repeat the treatment steps above.

14. To ensure that the improvements you've made are complete, perform the floor-to-ceiling eye roll (when the SUD is 2 or lower): Hold your head level and move your eyes down. Then begin tapping the gamut point as you move your eyes upward.

Complex Trauma with Anger Algorithm

1. Tune the Thought Field—that is, intentionally think about the traumatic event that produces such emotional distress in your life.

2. Rate your distress level at this moment, using the Subjective Units of Distress (SUD) scale. On this scale, 10 is the worst you could possibly feel, and 1 indicates absolutely no trace of upset. Write down the SUD rating.

3. Using two fingers of one hand, tap a spot at the beginning of the eyebrow, just above the bridge of the nose. Tap five times, firmly and gently, not nearly hard enough to bruise, but solidly enough to stimulate the energy flow in the system.

4. Tap five times under the eye, about an inch below the bottom of the eyeball, at the bottom of the center of the bony orbit, high on the cheek. Tap firmly, but not hard enough to cause pain.

5. Tap solidly five times under the arm, about four inches directly below the armpit, using rigid fingers. In men, this

spot is under the arm about even with the nipple. Women can locate this spot by tapping at about the center of the bra under the arm.

6. Tap the "collarbone point." To locate it, take two fingers of either hand and run them down the center of the throat to the top of the center collarbone notch. This is approximately even with the spot where a man would knot his tie. From there, move straight down an additional inch. Then move to the right one inch. Tap this point five times.

7. Tap the "little finger spot" five times. It is located on the inside tip of the finger, adjacent to the nail, and on the side of the finger next to the ring finger.

8. Tap the collarbone point five times again.

9. Take a second SUD rating and write it down. If it has decreased 2 or more points (which will be the case for most people), then continue with step 10 below. If there was no change, however, or if the change in the SUD was only 1 point, perform the correction for a psychological reversal, using the technique described in Chapter 4 (see page 84). Then repeat steps 1 through 9.

10. Perform the nine gamut treatments. Locate the gamut spot on the back of the hand, about an inch below the raised knuckles of the ring finger and little finger when making a fist. Begin tapping the gamut spot with two fingers of the opposite hand, about three to five times per second, and continue tapping while performing all nine steps below (tap five or six times for each of the nine gamut positions). It is very important to tap the gamut spot throughout all nine of these gamut treatments:

- Open the eyes.
- Close the eyes.
- Open the eyes and point them down and to the left.
- Point the eyes down and to the right.
- Whirl the eyes around in a circle in one direction.
- Whirl the eyes around in the opposite direction.
- Hum a few bars of any tune aloud (more than a single note; rest the eyes).
- Count aloud from one to five.
- Hum the tune again.

11. Tap the spot at the beginning of the eyebrow again. Tap five times, firmly and gently.
12. Tap under the eye five times again.
13. Tap solidly five times under the arm again.
14. Tap the collarbone point five times again.
15. Tap the little finger spot five times again.
16. Tap the collarbone point five times again.
17. Take still another SUD rating and write it down. If it has declined to 1 (which will happen with most people), move to step 18 below. But if it has decreased significantly yet is still not a 1, perform the mini PR correction as described in Chapter 4 (see page 85), and then repeat the treatment steps above.
18. To ensure that the improvements you've made are complete, perform the floor-to-ceiling eye roll (when the

SUD is 2 or lower): Hold your head level and move your eyes down. Then begin tapping the gamut point as you move your eyes upward.

Complex Trauma with Guilt Algorithm

1. Tune the Thought Field—that is, intentionally think about the traumatic event that produces such emotional distress in your life.

2. Rate your distress level at this moment, using the Subjective Units of Distress (SUD) scale. On this scale, 10 is the worst you could possibly feel, and 1 indicates absolutely no trace of upset. Write down the SUD rating.

3. Using two fingers of one hand, tap a spot at the beginning of the eyebrow, just above the bridge of the nose. Tap five times, firmly and gently, not nearly hard enough to bruise, but solidly enough to stimulate the energy flow in the system.

4. Tap five times under the eye, about an inch below the bottom of the eyeball, at the bottom of the center of the bony orbit, high on the cheek. Tap firmly, but not hard enough to cause pain.

5. Tap solidly five times under the arm, about four inches directly below the armpit, using rigid fingers. In men, this spot is under the arm about even with the nipple. Women can locate this spot by tapping at about the center of the bra under the arm.

6. Tap the "collarbone point." To locate it, take two fingers of either hand, and run them down the center of the throat to the top of the center collarbone notch. This is

approximately even with the spot where a man would knot his tie. From there, move straight down an additional inch. Then move to the right one inch. Tap this point five times.

7. Tap the "index finger spot" five times. It is located on the tip of the index (pointing) finger, on the side of that finger next to the thumb.

8. Tap the collarbone point five times again.

9. Take a second SUD rating and write it down. If it has decreased 2 or more points (which will be the case for most people), then continue with step 10 below. If there was no change, however, or if the change in the SUD was only 1 point, perform the correction for a psychological reversal, using the technique described in Chapter 4 (see page 84). Then repeat steps 1 through 9.

10. Perform the nine gamut treatments. Locate the gamut spot on the back of the hand, about an inch below the raised knuckles of the ring finger and little finger when making a fist. Begin tapping the gamut spot with two fingers of the opposite hand, about three to five times per second, and continue tapping while performing all nine steps below (tap five or six times for each of the nine gamut positions). It is very important to tap the gamut spot throughout all nine of these gamut treatments:

    - Open the eyes.
    - Close the eyes.
    - Open the eyes and point them down and to the left.
    - Point the eyes down and to the right.
    - Whirl the eyes around in a circle in one direction.

- Whirl the eyes around in the opposite direction.
- Hum a few bars of any tune aloud (more than a single note; rest the eyes).
- Count aloud from one to five.
- Hum the tune again.

11. Tap the spot at the beginning of the eyebrow again. Tap five times, firmly and gently.
12. Tap under the eye five times again.
13. Tap solidly five times under the arm again.
14. Tap the collarbone point five times again.
15. Tap the index finger spot five times again.
16. Tap the collarbone point five times again.
17. Take still another SUD rating and write it down. If it has declined to 1 (which will happen with most people), move to step 18 below. But if it has decreased significantly yet is still not a 1, perform the mini PR correction as described in Chapter 4 (see page 85), and then repeat the treatment steps above.
18. To ensure that the improvements you've made are complete, perform the floor-to-ceiling eye roll (when the SUD is 2 or lower): Hold your head level and move your eyes down. Then begin tapping the gamut spot as you move your eyes upward.

ANXIETY

If you have anxiety in your life, at least you're not alone. Some surveys have found that anxiety is the most common psychological disorder in the United States. It is so prevalent that many people accept it as an unwelcome fact of life. While it's true that anxiety often has no obvious trigger, it can also be attributed to factors such as the loss of a job or the illness of a family member. Even in cases like this, however, the anxiety is frequently out of proportion to the apparent cause; for example, a deadline at work may send your anxiety soaring far above what is warranted by the circumstances.

Remember, however, that no matter what you attribute your anxiety to, the key is collapsing the perturbations in the Thought Field that are responsible for it. Once those perturbations are eradicated, the anxiety will vanish as well.

Sometimes anxiety is accompanied by panic attacks. Panic is a sudden, intense onset of severe anxiety. For people who have never had a severe panic reaction, it is hard to imagine how disruptive and terrifying these episodes can be. Once they occur, they can dramatically affect how people live their lives, often leaving them fearful of having another panicky response, which makes them chronically anxious. They may consciously stay only in familiar and secure environments where such attacks are less likely to occur. In the most extreme cases, people become permanently homebound.

I recall a young mother who could not get more than six feet from her front door without having a severe panic attack. As a result, she was terrified about what might happen if her three-year-old son had a medical emergency that required an urgent trip to the hospital; she simply didn't think she'd be able to take him. Within a few minutes, after using the TFT algorithm, it was clear to her that she would be able to handle such an emergency.

The following algorithm is for "simple anxiety/stress." It will work for most people. If it doesn't get your SUD as low as you'd like, however, then use the algorithm for "complex anxiety/panic attack." Begin with the "first use" algorithm for complex anxiety, and then, if necessary, move on to one of the alternative algorithms.

Simple Anxiety/Stress Algorithm

1. Tune the Thought Field—that is, intentionally think about the anxiety that produces such emotional distress in your life.

2. Rate your distress level at this moment, using the Subjective Units of Distress (SUD) scale. On this scale, 10 is the worst you could possibly feel, and 1 indicates absolutely no trace of upset. Write down the SUD rating.

3. Using two fingers of one hand, tap five times under the eye, about an inch below the bottom of the center of the bony orbit, high on the cheek. Tap firmly, but not hard enough to cause pain.

4. Tap solidly five times under the arm, about four inches directly below the armpit, using rigid fingers. In men, this spot is under the arm about even with the nipple. Women can locate this spot by tapping at about the center of the bra under the arm.

5. Tap the "collarbone point." To locate it, take two fingers of either hand and run them down the center of the throat to the top of the center collarbone notch. This is approximately even with the spot where a man would knot his tie. From there, move straight down an additional inch. Then move to the right one inch. Tap this point five times.

6. Take a second SUD rating and write it down. If it has decreased 2 or more points (which will be the case for most people), then continue with step 7 below. If there was no change, however, or if the change in the SUD was only 1 point, perform the correction for a psychological reversal, using the technique described in Chapter 4 (see page 84). Then repeat steps 1 through 6.

7. Perform the nine gamut treatments. Locate the gamut spot on the back of the hand, about an inch below the raised knuckles of the ring finger and little finger when making a fist. Begin tapping the gamut spot with two fingers of the opposite hand, about three to five times per second, and continue tapping while performing all nine steps below (tap five or six times for each of the nine gamut positions). It is very important to tap the gamut spot throughout all nine of these gamut treatments:
   - Open the eyes.
   - Close the eyes.
   - Open the eyes and point them down and to the left.
   - Point the eyes down and to the right.
   - Whirl the eyes around in a circle in one direction.
   - Whirl the eyes around in the opposite direction.
   - Hum a few bars of any tune aloud (more than a single note; rest the eyes).
   - Count aloud from one to five.
   - Hum the tune again.
8. Tap five times under the eye again.
9. Tap five times under the arm again.
10. Tap the collarbone point five times again.
11. Take still another SUD rating and write it down. If it has declined to 1 (which will happen with most people), move to step 12 below. But if it has decreased significantly yet is still not a 1, perform the mini PR correction as described

in Chapter 4 (see page 85), and then repeat the treatment steps above.

12. To ensure that the improvements you've made are complete, perform the floor-to-ceiling eye roll (when the SUD is 2 or lower): Hold your head level and move your eyes down. Then begin tapping the gamut point as you move your eyes upward.

Complex Anxiety/Panic Attack Algorithm—First Use

1. Tune the Thought Field—that is, intentionally think about the anxiety that produces such emotional distress in your life.
2. Rate your distress level at this moment, using the Subjective Units of Distress (SUD) scale. On this scale, 10 is the worst you could possibly feel, and 1 indicates absolutely no trace of upset. Write down the SUD rating.
3. Using two fingers of one hand, tap a spot at the beginning of the eyebrow, just above the bridge of the nose. Tap five times, firmly but gently, not nearly hard enough to bruise, but solidly enough to stimulate the energy flow in the system.
4. Tap five times under the eye, about an inch below the bottom of the center of the bony orbit, high on the cheek. Tap firmly, but not hard enough to cause pain.
5. Tap solidly five times under the arm, about four inches directly below the armpit, using rigid fingers. In men, this spot is under the arm about even with the nipple. Women can locate this spot by tapping at about the center of the bra under the arm.

6. Tap the "collarbone point." To locate it, take two fingers of either hand and run them down the center of the throat to the top of the center collarbone notch. This is approximately even with the spot where a man would knot his tie. From there, move straight down an additional inch. Then move to the right one inch. Tap this point five times.

7. Take a second SUD rating and write it down. If it has decreased 2 or more points (which will be the case for most people), then continue with step 8 below. If there was no change, however, or if the change in the SUD was only 1 point, perform the correction for a psychological reversal, using the technique described in Chapter 4 (see page 84). Then repeat steps 1 through 7.

8. Perform the nine gamut treatments. Locate the gamut spot on the back of the hand, about an inch below the raised knuckles of the ring finger and little finger when making a fist. Begin tapping the gamut spot with two fingers of the opposite hand, about three to five times per second, and continue tapping while performing all nine steps below (tap five or six times for each of the nine gamut positions). It is very important to tap the gamut spot throughout all nine of these gamut treatments:

   - Open the eyes.
   - Close the eyes.
   - Open the eyes and point them down and to the left.
   - Point the eyes down and to the right.
   - Whirl the eyes around in a circle in one direction.
   - Whirl the eyes around in the opposite direction.
   - Hum a few bars of any tune aloud (more than a single note; rest the eyes).

- Count aloud from one to five.
- Hum the tune again.

9. Tap the spot at the beginning of the eyebrow five times again.
10. Tap five times under the eye again.
11. Tap five times under the arm again.
12. Tap the collarbone point five times again.
13. Take still another SUD rating and write it down. If it has declined to 1 (which will happen with most people), move to step 14 below. But if it has decreased significantly yet is still not a 1, perform the mini PR correction as described in Chapter 4 (page 85), and then repeat the treatment steps above.
14. To ensure that the improvements you've made are complete, perform the floor-to-ceiling eye roll (when the SUD is 2 or lower): Hold your head level and move your eyes down. Then begin tapping the gamut point as you move your eyes upward.

Complex Anxiety/Panic Attack Algorithm—Alternative 1

1. Tune the Thought Field—that is, intentionally think about the anxiety that produces such emotional distress in your life.
2. Rate your distress level at this moment, using the Subjective Units of Distress (SUD) scale. On this scale, 10 is the worst you could possibly feel, and 1 indicates absolutely no trace of upset. Write down the SUD rating.

3. Using two fingers of one hand, tap five times under the eye, about an inch below the bottom of the center of the bony orbit, high on the cheek. Tap firmly, but not hard enough to cause pain.

4. Tap solidly five times under the arm, about four inches directly below the armpit, using rigid fingers. In men, this spot is under the arm about even with the nipple. Women can locate this spot by tapping at about the center of the bra under the arm.

5. Tap a spot at the beginning of the eyebrow, just above the bridge of the nose. Tap five times, firmly but gently, not nearly hard enough to bruise, but solidly enough to stimulate the energy flow in the system.

6. Tap the "collarbone point." To locate it, take two fingers of either hand and run them down the center of the throat to the top of the center collarbone notch. This is approximately even with the spot where a man would knot his tie. From there, move straight down an additional inch. Then move to the right one inch. Tap this point five times.

7. Tap the "little finger spot" five times. It is located on the inside tip of the finger, adjacent to the nail, and on the side of the finger next to the ring finger.

8. Take a second SUD rating and write it down. If it has decreased 2 or more points (which will be the case for most people), then continue with step 9 below. If there was no change, however, or if the change in the SUD was only 1 point, perform the correction for a psychological reversal, using the technique described in Chapter 4 (see page 84). Then repeat steps 1 through 8.

9. Perform the nine gamut treatments. Locate the gamut spot on the back of the hand, about an inch below the raised

knuckles of the ring finger and little finger when making a fist. Begin tapping the gamut spot with two fingers of the opposite hand, about three to five times per second, and continue tapping while performing all nine steps below (tap five or six times for each of the nine gamut positions). It is very important to tap the gamut spot throughout all nine of these gamut treatments:

- Open the eyes.
- Close the eyes.
- Open the eyes and point them down and to the left.
- Point the eyes down and to the right.
- Whirl the eyes around in a circle in one direction.
- Whirl the eyes around in the opposite direction.
- Hum a few bars of any tune aloud (more than a single note; rest the eyes).
- Count aloud from one to five.
- Hum the tune again.

10. Tap five times under the eye again.
11. Tap five times under the arm again.
12. Tap the spot at the beginning of the eyebrow five times again.
13. Tap the collarbone point five times again.
14. Tap the little finger spot five times again.
15. Take still another SUD rating and write it down. If it has declined to 1 (which will happen with most people), move to step 16 below. But if it has decreased significantly yet is

still not a 1, perform the mini PR correction as described in Chapter 4 (see page 85), and then repeat the treatment steps above.

16. To ensure that the improvements you've made are complete, perform the floor-to-ceiling eye roll (when the SUD is 2 or lower): Hold your head level and move your eyes down. Then begin tapping the gamut point as you move your eyes upward.

Complex Anxiety/Panic Attack Algorithm—Alternative 2

1. Tune the Thought Field—that is, intentionally think about the anxiety that produces such emotional distress in your life.

2. Rate your distress level at this moment, using the Subjective Units of Distress (SUD) scale. On this scale, 10 is the worst you could possibly feel, and 1 indicates absolutely no trace of upset. Write down the SUD rating.

3. Using two fingers of one hand, tap solidly five times under the arm, about four inches directly below the armpit, using rigid fingers. In men, this spot is under the arm about even with the nipple. Women can locate this spot by tapping at about the center of the bra under the arm.

4. Tap five times under the eye, about an inch below the bottom of the center of the bony orbit, high on the cheek. Tap firmly, but not hard enough to cause pain.

5. Tap a spot at the beginning of the eyebrow, just above the bridge of the nose. Tap five times, firmly but gently, not nearly hard enough to bruise, but solidly enough to stimulate the energy flow in the system.

6. Tap the "collarbone point." To locate it, take two fingers of either hand and run them down the center of the throat to the top of the center collarbone notch. This is approximately even with the spot where a man would knot his tie. From there, move straight down an additional inch. Then move to the right one inch. Tap this point five times.

7. Tap the "little finger spot" five times. It is located on the inside tip of the finger, adjacent to the nail, and on the side of the finger next to the ring finger.

8. Take a second SUD rating and write it down. If it has decreased 2 or more points (which will be the case for most people), then continue with step 9 below. If there was no change, however, or if the change in the SUD was only 1 point, perform the correction for a psychological reversal, using the technique described in Chapter 4 (see page 84). Then repeat steps 1 through 8.

9. Perform the nine gamut treatments. Locate the gamut spot on the back of the hand, about an inch below the raised knuckles of the ring finger and little finger when making a fist. Begin tapping the gamut spot with two fingers of the opposite hand, about three to five times per second, and continue tapping while performing all nine steps below (tap five or six times for each of the nine gamut positions). It is very important to tap the gamut spot throughout all nine of these gamut treatments:

   - Open the eyes.
   - Close the eyes.
   - Open the eyes and point them down and to the left.
   - Point the eyes down and to the right.
   - Whirl the eyes around in a circle in one direction.

- Whirl the eyes around in the opposite direction.
- Hum a few bars of any tune aloud (more than a single note; rest the eyes).
- Count aloud from one to five.
- Hum the tune again.

10. Tap five times under the arm again.
11. Tap five times under the eye again.
12. Tap the spot at the beginning of the eyebrow five times again.
13. Tap the collarbone point five times again.
14. Tap the little finger spot five times again.
15. Take still another SUD rating and write it down. If it has declined to 1 (which will happen with most people), move to step 16 below. But if it has decreased significantly yet is still not a 1, perform the mini PR correction as described in Chapter 4 (see page 85), and then repeat the treatment steps above.
16. To ensure that the improvements you've made are complete, perform the floor-to-ceiling eye roll (when the SUD is 2 or lower): Hold your head level and move your eyes down. Then begin tapping the gamut point as you move your eyes upward.

Complex Anxiety/Panic Attack Algorithm—Alternative 3

1. Tune the Thought Field—that is, intentionally think about the anxiety that produces such emotional distress in your life.

2. Rate your distress level at this moment, using the Subjective Units of Distress (SUD) scale. On this scale, 10 is the worst you could possibly feel, and 1 indicates absolutely no trace of upset. Write down the SUD rating.

3. Using two fingers of one hand, tap a spot at the beginning of the eyebrow, just above the bridge of the nose. Tap five times, firmly but gently, not nearly hard enough to bruise, but solidly enough to stimulate the energy flow in the system.

4. Tap solidly five times under the arm, about four inches directly below the armpit, using rigid fingers. In men, this spot is under the arm about even with the nipple. Women can locate this spot by tapping at about the center of the bra under the arm.

5. Tap five times under the eye, about an inch below the bottom of the center of the bony orbit, high on the cheek. Tap firmly, but not hard enough to cause pain.

6. Take a second SUD rating and write it down. If it has decreased 2 or more points (which will be the case for most people), then continue with step 7 below. If there was no change, however, or if the change in the SUD was only 1 point, perform the correction for a psychological reversal, using the technique described in Chapter 4 (see page 84). Then repeat steps 1 through 6.

7. Perform the nine gamut treatments. Locate the gamut spot on the back of the hand, about an inch below the raised knuckles of the ring finger and little finger when making a fist. Begin tapping the gamut spot with two fingers of the opposite hand, about three to five times per second, and continue tapping while performing all nine steps below (tap five or six times for each of the nine gamut positions).

It is very important to tap the gamut spot throughout all nine of these gamut treatments:

- Open the eyes.
- Close the eyes.
- Open the eyes and point them down and to the left.
- Point the eyes down and to the right.
- Whirl the eyes around in a circle in one direction.
- Whirl the eyes around in the opposite direction.
- Hum a few bars of any tune aloud (more than a single note; rest the eyes).
- Count aloud from one to five.
- Hum the tune again.

8. Tap the spot at the beginning of the eyebrow five times again.
9. Tap five times under the arm again.
10. Tap five times under the eye again.
11. Take still another SUD rating and write it down. If it has declined to 1 (which will happen with most people), move to step 12 below. But if it has decreased significantly yet is still not a 1, perform the mini PR correction as described in Chapter 4 (see page 85), and then repeat the treatment steps above.
12. To ensure that the improvements you've made are complete, perform the floor-to-ceiling eye roll (when the SUD is 2 or lower): Hold your head level and move your eyes down. Then begin tapping the gamut point as you move your eyes upward.

Complex Anxiety/Panic Attack Algorithm—Alternative 4

1. Tune the Thought Field—that is, intentionally think about the anxiety that produces such emotional distress in your life.

2. Rate your distress level at this moment, using the Subjective Units of Distress (SUD) scale. On this scale, 10 is the worst you could possibly feel, and 1 indicates absolutely no trace of upset. Write down the SUD rating.

3. Using two fingers of one hand, tap five times under the eye, about an inch below the bottom of the center of the bony orbit, high on the cheek. Tap firmly, but not hard enough to cause pain.

4. Tap a spot at the beginning of the eyebrow, just above the bridge of the nose. Tap five times, firmly but gently, not nearly hard enough to bruise, but solidly enough to stimulate the energy flow in the system.

5. Tap solidly five times under the arm, about four inches directly below the armpit, using rigid fingers. In men, this spot is under the arm about even with the nipple. Women can locate this spot by tapping at about the center of the bra under the arm.

6. Tap the "little finger spot" five times. It is located on the inside tip of the finger, adjacent to the nail, and on the side of the finger next to the ring finger.

7. Take a second SUD rating and write it down. If it has decreased 2 or more points (which will be the case for most people), then continue with step 8 below. If there was no change, however, or if the change in the SUD was only 1 point, perform the correction for a psychological reversal,

using the technique described in Chapter 4 (see page 84). Then repeat steps 1 through 7.

8. Perform the nine gamut treatments. Locate the gamut spot on the back of the hand, about an inch below the raised knuckles of the ring finger and little finger when making a fist. Begin tapping the gamut spot with two fingers of the opposite hand, about three to five times per second, and continue tapping while performing all nine steps below (tap five or six times for each of the nine gamut positions). It is very important to tap the gamut spot throughout all nine of these gamut treatments:

   - Open the eyes.
   - Close the eyes.
   - Open the eyes and point them down and to the left.
   - Point the eyes down and to the right.
   - Whirl the eyes around in a circle in one direction.
   - Whirl the eyes around in the opposite direction.
   - Hum a few bars of any tune aloud (more than a single note; rest the eyes).
   - Count aloud from one to five.
   - Hum the tune again.

9. Tap five times under the eye again.
10. Tap the spot at the beginning of the eyebrow five times again.
11. Tap five times under the arm again.
12. Tap the little finger spot five times again.

13. Take still another SUD rating and write it down. If it has declined to 1 (which will happen with most people), move to step 14 below. But if it has decreased significantly yet is still not a 1, perform the mini PR correction as described in Chapter 4 (see page 85), and then repeat the treatment steps above.

14. To ensure that the improvements you've made are complete, perform the floor-to-ceiling eye roll (when the SUD is 2 or lower): Hold your head level and move your eyes down. Then begin tapping the gamut point as you move your eyes upward.

Complex Anxiety/Panic Attack Algorithm—Alternative 5

1. Tune the Thought Field—that is, intentionally think about the anxiety that produces such emotional distress in your life.

2. Rate your distress level at this moment, using the Subjective Units of Distress (SUD) scale. On this scale, 10 is the worst you could possibly feel, and 1 indicates absolutely no trace of upset. Write down the SUD rating.

3. Tap the "collarbone point." To locate it, take two fingers of either hand and run them down the center of the throat to the top of the center collarbone notch. This is approximately even with the spot where a man would knot his tie. From there, move straight down an additional inch. Then move to the right one inch. Tap this point five times.

4. Tap five times under the eye, about an inch below the bottom of the center of the bony orbit, high on the cheek. Tap firmly, but not hard enough to cause pain.

5. Tap solidly five times under the arm, about four inches directly below the armpit, using rigid fingers. In men, this spot is under the arm about even with the nipple. Women can locate this spot by tapping at about the center of the bra under the arm.

6. Take a second SUD rating and write it down. If it has decreased 2 or more points (which will be the case for most people), then continue with step 7 below. If there was no change, however, or if the change in the SUD was only 1 point, perform the correction for a psychological reversal, using the technique described in Chapter 4 (see page 84). Then repeat steps 1 through 6.

7. Perform the nine gamut treatments. Locate the gamut spot on the back of the hand, about an inch below the raised knuckles of the ring finger and little finger when making a fist. Begin tapping the gamut spot with two fingers of the opposite hand, about three to five times per second, and continue tapping while performing all nine steps below (tap five or six times for each of the nine gamut positions). It is very important to tap the gamut spot throughout all nine of these gamut treatments:

   - Open the eyes.
   - Close the eyes.
   - Open the eyes and point them down and to the left.
   - Point the eyes down and to the right.
   - Whirl the eyes around in a circle in one direction.
   - Whirl the eyes around in the opposite direction.
   - Hum a few bars of any tune aloud (more than a single note; rest the eyes).

- Count aloud from one to five.
- Hum the tune again.

8. Tap the collarbone point five times again.
9. Tap five times under the eye again.
10. Tap five times under the arm again.
11. Take still another SUD rating and write it down. If it has declined to 1 (which will happen with most people), move to step 12 below. But if it has decreased significantly yet is still not a 1, perform the mini PR correction as described in Chapter 4 (see page 85), and then repeat the treatments above.
12. To ensure that the improvements you've made are complete, perform the floor-to-ceiling eye roll (when the SUD is 2 or lower): Hold your head level and move your eyes down. Then begin tapping the gamut point as you move your eyes upward.

ADDICTIVE URGES

Addictive urges are a dominating force in the lives of many millions of people. But whether you're addicted to nicotine, heroin, alcohol, or food, Thought Field Therapy can help your problem in minutes. Even if you've been a smoker for decades, or have failed dozens of diets in an attempt to control your intake of food, a brief algorithm can put the problem to rest for good.

Over the years, as the prevalence of addictions has soared to an epidemic in America, I've recognized that addictions are a reaction to anxiety (I've confirmed this through Causal Diagnosis). All addictions, in fact, are addictions to a substance or activity to mask this anxiety. However, addiction is an inappropriate way to deal with anxiety in that it only attempts to cover it up but doesn't actually eradicate it. In order to treat an addiction, the underlying anxiety must be treated.

So, for example, when your stress levels at work are particularly high, do you feel like lighting up a cigarette? Or do you reach for a candy bar? The overpowering urge to smoke or to eat is triggered by anxiety and by the desire to find false comfort and calmness through food or any other addiction. Remember, however, food or drugs don't really ease the anxiety itself, although they may appear to; they only cover it up like a blanket, actually making addiction more likely and worsening the anxiety. As these substances seem to provide a tranquilizing effect, the addictive urge subconsciously gets reinforced.

One of the first clients I treated for addictive urges was a woman I'll call Anne. Her addiction was to Snickers candy bars, and at least three times a day, she would grab one from her purse and munch away. They were always there for "emergencies," she said, and to her mind, they were the perfect tranquilizer. Although her doctor had advised her to lose weight and to cut excess fat and calories from her diet, Anne just wasn't able to stop giving in to her candy cravings. After a single treatment with a TFT algorithm, however, all of that changed. Her SUD (reflecting her desire for a Snickers bar) plummeted from 9 to 1. I have kept in touch with Anne, and her addiction has not returned for years.

Just how powerful are these addictive urges? Consider that most smokers who survive a heart attack—or who undergo coronary bypass surgery—continue to smoke. Imagine looking death in the eye and getting a second chance at life, and yet continuing with the behavior that may have been largely responsible for the health problems you experienced!

I've often told the story about the U.S. soldiers who fought in the Vietnam War. Some of them turned to heroin and other illegal drugs to smother their reality-based anxiety. As word drifted back to the States about heroin use among GIs, there was a fear that America would have to deal with severe drug-addiction problems as the soldiers came home. But that wasn't the case at all. Once the returnees left the anxiety of combat behind them (obviously, the source of their anxiety was outside of themselves), most of them simply stopped using these hard drugs. They no longer felt the need for them, and the physiological component of addiction seemed rather insignificant once the source of their anxiety was gone. I'm convinced that addiction is primarily a psychological problem, not a physical one.

By treating the addictive urges in your life with the algorithms that follow, you won't be masking or covering them up—you'll be eradicating them at their root cause.

Begin with the "first use" algorithm below, which works for most people in eliminating their addictive urges. But if you don't have success with it, move on to the "alternative algorithms," which are more effective for some individuals. Use these algorithms when your addictive urge is particularly strong.

Addictive Urge Algorithm—First Use

1. Tune the Thought Field—that is, intentionally think about the addictive urge you want to treat.

2. Rate the intensity of your addictive urge at this moment, using the Subjective Units of Distress (SUD) scale. On this scale, 10 is the most intense it could possibly be, and 1 indicates absolutely no trace of it. Write down the SUD rating.

3. Using two fingers of one hand, tap five times under the eye, about an inch below the bottom of the center of the bony orbit, high on the cheek. Tap firmly, but not hard enough to cause pain.

4. Tap solidly five times under the arm, about four inches directly below the armpit, using rigid fingers. In men, this spot is under the arm about even with the nipple. Women can locate this spot by tapping at about the center of the bra under the arm.

5. Tap the "collarbone point." To locate it, take two fingers of either hand and run them down the center of the throat to the top of the center collarbone notch. This is approximately even with the spot where a man would knot his tie. From there, move straight down an additional inch. Then move to the right one inch. Tap this point five times.

6. Take a second SUD rating and write it down. If it has decreased 2 or more points (which will be the case for most people), then continue with step 7 below. If there was no change, however, or if the change in the SUD was only 1 point, perform the correction for a psychological reversal, using the technique described in Chapter 4 (see page 84). Then repeat steps 1 through 6.

7. Perform the nine gamut treatments. Locate the gamut spot on the back of the hand, about an inch below the raised knuckles of the ring finger and little finger when making a fist. Begin tapping the gamut spot with two fingers of the opposite hand, about three to five times per second, and continue tapping while performing all nine steps below (tap five or six times for each of the nine gamut positions). It is very important to tap the gamut spot throughout all nine of these gamut treatments:

   - Open the eyes.
   - Close the eyes.
   - Open the eyes and point them down and to the left.

- Point the eyes down and to the right.
- Whirl the eyes around in a circle in one direction.
- Whirl the eyes around in the opposite direction.
- Hum a few bars of any tune aloud (more than a single note; rest the eyes).
- Count aloud from one to five.
- Hum the tune again.

8. Tap five times under the eye again.
9. Tap five times under the arm again.
10. Tap the collarbone point five times again.
11. Take still another SUD rating and write it down. If it has declined to 1 (which will happen with most people), move to step 12 below. But if it has decreased significantly yet is still not a 1, perform the mini PR correction as described in Chapter 4 (see page 85), and then repeat the treatment steps above.
12. To ensure that the improvements you've made are complete, perform the floor-to-ceiling eye roll (when the SUD is 2 or lower): Hold your head level and move your eyes down. Then begin tapping the gamut point as you move your eyes upward.

Addictive Urge Algorithm—Alternative 1

1. Tune the Thought Field—that is, intentionally think about the addictive urge you want to treat.
2. Rate the intensity of your addictive urge at this moment, using the Subjective Units of Distress (SUD) scale. On

this scale, 10 is the most intense it could possibly be, and 1 indicates absolutely no trace of it. Write down the SUD rating.

3. Tap the "collarbone point." To locate it, take two fingers of either hand and run them down the center of the throat to the top of the center collarbone notch. This is approximately even with the spot where a man would knot his tie. From there, move straight down an additional inch. Then move to the right one inch. Tap this point five times.

4. Using two fingers of one hand, tap five times under the eye, about an inch below the bottom of the center of the bony orbit, high on the cheek. Tap firmly, but not hard enough to cause pain.

5. Tap the collarbone point five times again.

6. Take a second SUD rating and write it down. If it has decreased 2 or more points (which will be the case for most people), then continue with step 7 below. If there was no change, however, or if the change in the SUD was only 1 point, perform the correction for a psychological reversal, using the technique described in Chapter 4 (see page 84). Then repeat steps 1 through 6.

7. Perform the nine gamut treatments. Locate the gamut spot on the back of the hand, about an inch below the raised knuckles of the ring finger and little finger when making a fist. Begin tapping the gamut spot with two fingers of the opposite hand, about three to five times per second, and continue tapping while performing all nine steps below (tap five or six times for each of the nine gamut positions). It is very important to tap the gamut spot throughout all nine of these gamut treatments:

   - Open the eyes.

- Close the eyes.
- Open the eyes and point them down and to the left.
- Point the eyes down and to the right.
- Whirl the eyes around in a circle in one direction.
- Whirl the eyes around in the opposite direction.
- Hum a few bars of any tune aloud (more than a single note; rest the eyes).
- Count aloud from one to five.
- Hum the tune again.

8. Tap the collarbone point five times again.
9. Tap five times under the eye again.
10. Tap the collarbone point five times again.
11. Take still another SUD rating and write it down. If it has declined to 1 (which will happen with most people), move to step 12 below. But if it has decreased significantly yet is still not a 1, perform the mini PR correction as described in Chapter 4 (see page 85), and then repeat the treatment steps above.
12. To ensure that the improvements you've made are complete, perform the floor-to-ceiling eye roll (when the SUD is 2 or lower): Hold your head level and move your eyes down. Then begin tapping the gamut point as you move your eyes upward.

Addictive Urge Algorithm—Alternative 2

1. Tune the Thought Field—that is, intentionally think about the addictive urge you want to treat.

2. Rate the intensity of your addictive urge at this moment, using the Subjective Units of Distress (SUD) scale. On this scale, 10 is the most intense it could possibly be, and 1 indicates absolutely no trace of it. Write down the SUD rating.

3. Tap solidly five times under the arm, about four inches directly below the armpit, using rigid fingers. In men, this spot is under the arm about even with the nipple. Women can locate this spot by tapping at about the center of the bra under the arm.

4. Using two fingers of one hand, tap five times under the eye, about an inch below the bottom of the center of the bony orbit, high on the cheek. Tap firmly, but not hard enough to cause pain.

5. Tap the "collarbone point." To locate it, take two fingers of either hand, and run them down the center of the throat to the top of the center collarbone notch. This is approximately even with the spot where a man would knot his tie. From there, move straight down an additional inch. Then move to the right one inch. Tap this point five times.

6. Take a second SUD rating and write it down. If it has decreased 2 or more points (which will be the case for most people), then continue with step 7 below. If there was no change, however, or if the change in the SUD was only 1 point, perform the correction for a psychological reversal, using the technique described in Chapter 4 (see page 84). Then repeat steps 1 through 6.

7. Perform the nine gamut treatments. Locate the gamut spot on the back of the hand, about an inch below the raised knuckles of the ring finger and little finger when making a fist. Begin tapping the gamut spot with two fingers of the opposite hand, about three to five times per second, and

continue tapping while performing all nine steps below (tap five or six times for each of the nine gamut positions). It is very important to tap the gamut spot throughout all nine of these gamut treatments:

- Open the eyes.
- Close the eyes.
- Open the eyes and point them down and to the left.
- Point the eyes down and to the right.
- Whirl the eyes around in a circle in one direction.
- Whirl the eyes around in the opposite direction.
- Hum a few bars of any tune aloud (more than a single note; rest the eyes).
- Count aloud from one to five.
- Hum the tune again.

8. Tap five times under the arm again.
9. Tap under the eye five times again.
10. Tap the collarbone point five times again.
11. Take still another SUD rating and write it down. If it has declined to 1 (which will happen with most people), move to step 12 below. But if it has decreased significantly yet is still not a 1, perform the mini PR correction as described in Chapter 4 (see page 85), and then repeat the treatment steps above.
12. To ensure that the improvements you've made are complete, perform the floor-to-ceiling eye roll (when the SUD is 2 or lower): Hold your head level and move your

eyes down. Then begin tapping the gamut point as you move your eyes upward.

PHOBIAS

A phobia is a persistent fear without a rational basis, typically related to a harmless object or situation. Ironically, most people who have these phobias understand quite well how unrealistic their fear is, which makes them feel even more foolish and ashamed, and contributes further to their emotional distress. They know they shouldn't be afraid, but they simply can't rid themselves of it.

Most mainstream psychologists actually believe that phobias can't be cured. That has been devastating news for phobics whose fears have disrupted their careers, hurt their relationships, and sabotaged their ability to enjoy life. For many years, that was terrible news for me as well. I grew up in foster homes, where I suffered in silence dealing with fears of heights, tunnels, and speaking in front of others. If only I had known the phobia algorithm back then, it could have saved me from plenty of agony.

Some time ago, I met a woman at the base of the aerial tram in Palm Springs, California, which travels thousands of feet to the top of San Jacinto Mountain. Although she wanted to ride on the tram, she was petrified of heights, and so she just stood there, unable to take the few steps necessary to board the gondola. With her permission, I treated her with a TFT algorithm on the spot—and it worked. Within minutes, she said she felt fine. Her SUD, she said, had plummeted to 1. She and I boarded the tram, and I rode next to her to the top of the mountain. She clearly enjoyed the ride, free of the fear that had caused trembling, heart palpitations, and a flushed face just minutes earlier.

The algorithms that follow can produce the same kind of instantaneous, painless healing of your own fears. There are two phobia algorithms. One is for most phobias and fears. It is effective for fear of heights, bridges, cats, dogs, bugs, snakes, needles, dentists, mice, horses, water, closed spaces, public speaking, and all other phobias except the three mentioned below (public speaking, by the way, is the most common fear, but can often be rapidly resolved with this algorithm). The other algorithm is for three specific phobias—spiders, claustrophobia, and air turbulence (in flight). It is a particularly effective treatment for these conditions.

During an appearance I made on a radio talk show, a caller described her intense fear of spiders. Just the sight of a spider, she said, would leave her shaking and feeling faint. On the SUD scale, she said she was a 10 at that moment. Then I guided her through the phobia algorithm. After this brief treatment lasting only two minutes, she reported that her SUD reading had plummeted to a 1.

The radio show continued for almost another hour. Just before it ended, the woman called back. There was genuine excitement in her voice. She said that she had phoned in again because while sitting on her couch, she noticed that a spider had begun crawling on her lap. An hour earlier, that might have been one of the most terrifying moments of her life. But she described feeling no fear at all as she calmly watched the spider make its way across her lap and back onto the couch. Her SUD score of 1 clearly correlated with the dramatic elimination of her fear.

Most Phobias

1. Tune the Thought Field—that is, intentionally think about the phobia that you are treating.
2. Using the Subjective Units of Distress (SUD) scale, determine how upset you feel at this moment when thinking about the phobia. On this scale, 10 is the worst

you could possibly feel, and 1 indicates absolutely no trace of upset. Write down the SUD rating.

3. Using two fingers of one hand, tap five times under the eye, about an inch below the bottom of the center of the bony orbit, high on the cheek. Tap firmly, but not hard enough to cause pain.

4. Tap solidly five times under the arm, about four inches directly below the armpit, using rigid fingers. In men, this spot is under the arm about even with the nipple. Women can locate this spot by tapping at about the center of the bra under the arm.

5. Tap the "collarbone point." To locate it, take two fingers of either hand and run them down the center of the throat to the top of the center collarbone notch. This is approximately even with the spot where a man would knot his tie. From there, move straight down an additional inch. Then move to the right one inch. Tap this point five times.

6. Take a second SUD rating and write it down. If it has decreased 2 or more points (which will be the case for most people), then continue with step 7 below. If there was no change, however, or if the change in the SUD was only 1 point, perform the correction for a psychological reversal, using the technique described in Chapter 4 (see page 84). Then repeat steps 1 through 6.

7. Perform the nine gamut treatments. Locate the gamut spot on the back of the hand, about an inch below the raised knuckles of the ring finger and little finger when making a fist. Begin tapping the gamut spot with two fingers of the opposite hand, about three to five times per second, and continue tapping while performing all nine steps below

(tap five or six times for each of the nine gamut positions). It is very important to tap the gamut spot throughout all nine of these gamut treatments:

- Open the eyes.
- Close the eyes.
- Open the eyes and point them down and to the left.
- Point the eyes down and to the right.
- Whirl the eyes around in a circle in one direction.
- Whirl the eyes around in the opposite direction.
- Hum a few bars of any tune aloud (more than a single note; rest the eyes).
- Count aloud from one to five.
- Hum the tune again.

8. Tap five times under the eye again.
9. Tap five times under the arm again.
10. Tap the collarbone point five times again.
11. Take still another SUD rating and write it down. If it has declined to 1 (which will happen with most people), move to step 12 below. But if it has decreased significantly yet is still not a 1, perform the mini PR correction as described in Chapter 4 (see page 85), and then repeat the treatment steps above.
12. To ensure that the improvements you've made are complete, perform the floor-to-ceiling eye roll (when the SUD is 2 or lower): Hold your head level and move your eyes down. Then begin tapping the gamut point as you move your eyes upward.

Fear of Spiders, Claustrophobia, and Turbulence

1. Tune the Thought Field—that is, intentionally think about the phobia that you are treating.

2. Using the Subjective Units of Distress (SUD) scale, determine how upset you feel at this moment when thinking about the phobia. On this scale, 10 is the worst you could possibly feel, and 1 indicates absolutely no trace of upset. Write down the SUD rating.

3. Tap solidly five times under the arm, about four inches directly below the armpit, using rigid fingers. In men, this spot is under the arm about even with the nipple. Women can locate this spot by tapping at about the center of the bra under the arm.

4. Using two fingers of one hand, tap five times under the eye, about an inch below the bottom of the center of the bony orbit, high on the cheek. Tap firmly, but not hard enough to cause pain.

5. Tap the "collarbone point." To locate it, take two fingers of either hand and run them down the center of the throat to the top of the center collarbone notch. This is approximately even with the spot where a man would knot his tie. From there, move straight down an additional inch. Then move to the right one inch. Tap this point five times.

6. Take a second SUD rating and write it down. If it has decreased 2 or more points (which will be the case for most people), then continue with step 7 below. If there was no change, however, or if the change in the SUD was only 1 point, perform the correction for a psychological reversal, using the technique described in Chapter 4 (see page 84). Then repeat steps 1 through 6.

7. Perform the nine gamut treatments. Locate the gamut spot on the back of the hand, about an inch below the raised knuckles of the ring finger and little finger when making a fist. Begin tapping the gamut spot with two fingers of the opposite hand, about three to five times per second, and continue tapping while performing all nine steps below (tap five or six times for each of the nine gamut positions). It is very important to tap the gamut spot throughout all nine of these gamut treatments:

   - Open the eyes.
   - Close the eyes.
   - Open the eyes and point them down and to the left.
   - Point the eyes down and to the right.
   - Whirl the eyes around in a circle in one direction.
   - Whirl the eyes around in the opposite direction.
   - Hum a few bars of any tune aloud (more than a single note; rest the eyes).
   - Count aloud from one to five.
   - Hum the tune again.

8. Tap five times under the arm again.
9. Tap under the eye five times again.
10. Tap the collarbone point five times again.
11. Take still another SUD rating and write it down. If it has declined to 1 (which will happen with most people), move to step 12 below. But if it has decreased significantly yet is still not a 1, perform the mini PR correction as described in Chapter 4 (see page 85), and then repeat the treatments above.

12. To ensure that the improvements you've made are complete, perform the floor-to-ceiling eye roll (when the SUD is 2 or lower): Hold your head level and move your eyes down. Then begin tapping the gamut point as you move your eyes upward.

DEPRESSION

Everyone gets the blues from time to time. But depression is quite a different phenomenon. It produces a powerful and chronic pall of crippling sadness, suffering, and hopelessness that makes it virtually impossible to enjoy life. Depressed people have difficulty concentrating, feel lethargic and fatigued, withdraw from family and friends, and lose interest in pleasurable activities.

Depression occurs about twice as frequently in women as in men. But the following algorithm is effective for the overwhelming majority of people of both sexes. Nevertheless, here is an important caveat: while the algorithm is helpful, *you also need to be under the care of a mental health professional if you are depressed.* That's because depression increases the risk of suicide. Suicidal talk or thoughts represent a medical and psychological emergency.

Depression Algorithm

1. Tune the Thought Field—that is, intentionally think about the depression.

2. Rate the severity of your depression at this moment, using the Subjective Units of Distress (SUD) scale. On this scale, 10 is the worst you could possibly feel, and 1 indicates absolutely no trace of upset. Write down the SUD rating.

3. Locate the gamut spot on the back of the hand, about an inch below the raised knuckles of the ring finger and little finger when making a fist. Tap this gamut spot thirty times, using two fingers of the opposite hand.

4. Tap the "collarbone point." To locate it, take two fingers of either hand, and run them down the center of the throat to the top of the center collarbone notch. This is approximately even with the spot where a man would knot his tie. From there, move straight down an additional inch. Then move to the right one inch. Tap this point five times.

5. Take a second SUD rating and write it down. If it has decreased 2 or more points (which will be the case for most people), then continue with step 6 below. If there was no change, however, or if the change in the SUD was only 1 point, perform the correction for a psychological reversal, using the technique described in Chapter 4 (see page 84). Then repeat steps 1 through 5.

6. Perform the nine gamut treatments. Locate the gamut spot on the back of the hand (see step 3 above). Then begin tapping the gamut spot with two fingers of the opposite hand, about three to five times per second, and continue tapping while performing all nine steps below (tap five or six times for each of the nine gamut positions). It is very important to tap the gamut spot throughout all nine of these gamut treatments:

   - Open the eyes.
   - Close the eyes.
   - Open the eyes and point them down and to the left.
   - Point the eyes down and to the right.
   - Whirl the eyes around in a circle in one direction.

- Whirl the eyes around in the opposite direction.
- Hum a few bars of any tune aloud (more than a single note; rest the eyes).
- Count aloud from one to five.
- Hum the tune again.

7. Tap the gamut spot thirty times again.
8. Tap the collarbone point five times again.
9. Take still another SUD rating and write it down. If it has declined to 1 (which will happen with most people), move to step 10 below. But if it has decreased significantly yet is still not a 1, perform the mini PR correction as described in Chapter 4 (see page 85), and then repeat the treatment steps above.
10. To ensure that the improvements you've made are complete, perform the floor-to-ceiling eye roll (when the SUD is 2 or lower): Hold your head level and move your eyes down. Then begin tapping the gamut point as you move your eyes upward.

ANGER AND RAGE

Anger can be a crippling emotion, and one that many people handle poorly. When it becomes chronic—unresolved anger with a spouse, a misbehaving adolescent, or an overly demanding boss, for example—it can put your physical health at risk, too, increasing blood pressure, releasing stress hormones, and escalating the risk of heart attacks.

Women in particular are often taught to suppress their anger rather than express it. But burying anger can lead to everything from depression to physical ailments. At the other extreme, anger may trigger shouting and screaming, which does nothing to resolve the underlying emotion and often simply escalates the level of anger. It is much healthier to calm the emotion, and *nothing* can accomplish that more quickly and effectively than Thought Field Therapy.

Below you will find two algorithms—one for anger and the second for rage. Choose the first one for most situations in which anger has pervaded your life. Rage is a more intense, all-consuming anger in which an individual may even lose control and express that rage with physical abuse of a spouse or child. As a general guideline, begin with the anger algorithm; if it isn't completely effective, then try the rage algorithm.

Anger Algorithm

1. Tune the Thought Field—that is, intentionally think about the anger that you are treating.

2. Rate the severity of your anger at this moment, using the Subjective Units of Distress (SUD) scale. On this scale, 10 is the worst you could possibly feel, and 1 indicates absolutely no trace of upset. Write down the SUD rating.

3. Tap the "little finger spot" five times. It is located on the inside tip of the finger, adjacent to the nail, and on the side of the finger next to the ring finger.

4. Tap the "collarbone point." To locate it, take two fingers of either hand and run them down the center of the throat to the top of the center collarbone notch. This is approximately even with the spot where a man would knot his tie. From there, move straight down an additional inch. Then move to the right one inch. Tap this point five times.

5. Take a second SUD rating and write it down. If it has decreased 2 or more points (which will be the case for most people), then continue with step 6 below. If there was no change, however, or if the change in the SUD was only 1 point, perform the correction for a psychological reversal, using the technique described in Chapter 4 (see page 84). Then repeat steps 1 through 5.

6. Perform the nine gamut treatments. Locate the gamut spot on the back of the hand, about an inch below the raised knuckles of the ring finger and little finger when making a fist. Begin tapping the gamut spot with two fingers of the opposite hand, about three to five times per second, and continue tapping while performing all nine steps below (tap five or six times for each of the nine gamut positions). It is very important to tap the gamut spot throughout all nine of these gamut treatments:

   - Open the eyes.
   - Close the eyes.
   - Open the eyes and point them down and to the left.
   - Point the eyes down and to the right.
   - Whirl the eyes around in a circle in one direction.
   - Whirl the eyes around in the opposite direction.
   - Hum a few bars of any tune aloud (more than a single note; rest the eyes).
   - Count aloud from one to five.
   - Hum the tune again.

7. Tap the little finger spot five times again.

8. Tap the collarbone point five times again.

9. Take still another SUD rating and write it down. If it has declined to 1 (which will happen with most people), move to step 10 below. But if it has decreased significantly yet is still not a 1, perform the mini PR correction as described in Chapter 4 (see page 85), and then repeat the treatment steps above.

10. To ensure that the improvements you've made are complete, perform the floor-to-ceiling eye roll (when the SUD is 2 or lower): Hold your head level and move your eyes down. Then begin tapping the gamut point as you move your eyes upward.

Rage Algorithm

1. Tune the Thought Field—that is, intentionally think about the rage that produces such emotional distress in your life.

2. Rate the intensity of your rage at this moment, using the Subjective Units of Distress (SUD) scale. On this scale, 10 is the worst you could possibly feel, and 1 indicates absolutely no trace of rage. Write down the SUD rating.

3. Using two fingers of one hand, tap a spot on the outside edge of the eye. Tap five times, firmly and gently, but not nearly hard enough to bruise.

4. Tap the "collarbone point." To locate it, take two fingers of either hand and run them down the center of the throat to the top of the center collarbone notch. This is approximately even with the spot where a man would knot his tie. From there, move straight down an additional

inch. Then move to the right one inch. Tap this point five times.

5. Take a second SUD rating and write it down. If it has decreased 2 or more points (which will be the case for most people), then continue with step 6 below. If there was no change, however, or if the change in the SUD was only 1 point, perform the correction for a psychological reversal, using the technique described in Chapter 4 (see page 84). Then repeat steps 1 through 5.

6. Perform the nine gamut treatments. Locate the gamut spot on the back of the hand, about an inch below the raised knuckles of the ring finger and little finger when making a fist. Begin tapping the gamut spot with two fingers of the opposite hand, about three to five times per second, and continue tapping while performing all nine steps below (tap five or six times for each of the nine gamut positions). It is very important to tap the gamut spot throughout all nine of these gamut treatments:

    - Open the eyes.
    - Close the eyes.
    - Open the eyes and point them down and to the left.
    - Point the eyes down and to the right.
    - Whirl the eyes around in a circle in one direction.
    - Whirl the eyes around in the opposite direction.
    - Hum a few bars of any tune aloud (more than a single note; rest the eyes).
    - Count aloud from one to five.
    - Hum the tune again.

7. Tap the outside edge of the eye five times again.

8. Tap the collarbone point five times again.

9. Take still another SUD rating and write it down. If it has declined to 1 (which will happen with most people), move to step 10 below. But if it has decreased significantly yet is still not a 1, perform the mini PR correction as described in Chapter 4 (see page 85), and then repeat the treatment steps above.

10. To ensure that the improvements you've made are complete, perform the floor-to-ceiling eye roll (when the SUD is 2 or lower): Hold your head level and move your eyes down. Then begin tapping the gamut point as you move your eyes upward.

OBSESSIONS

Obsessions are repetitive thoughts or impulses generated by anxiety. To decrease that anxiety, people often develop and rely on compulsions (repetitive behaviors or actions). Hence the term *obsessive-compulsive disorder* (OCD) to describe this common condition. OCD is actually an addiction to certain anxiety-*masking* behaviors.

People with OCD may check again and again whether they've turned off the flame on the stove or whether they've locked the front door, seemingly unable to calm their anxiety over whether they've really checked. People with obsessions may also worry that they are catching diseases from objects or from other people, and consequently they'll wash their hands repeatedly.

The following algorithms can treat obsession (and OCD). They should be used when your obsessive urge is high. Begin with the "first use" algorithm. Then, if necessary, move on to one of the alternative algorithms.

Obsession (OCD) Algorithm—First Use

1. Tune the Thought Field—that is, intentionally think about the obsession that you are treating.
2. Using the Subjective Units of Distress (SUD) scale, rate the intensity of your urge to engage in the obsessive behavior at this moment. On this scale, 10 is the worst you could possibly feel, and 1 indicates absolutely no trace of upset. Write down the SUD rating.
3. Tap the "collarbone point." To locate it, take two fingers of either hand and run them down the center of the throat to the top of the center collarbone notch. This is approximately even with the spot where a man would knot his tie. From there, move straight down an additional inch. Then move to the right one inch. Tap this point five times.
4. Tap five times under the eye, about an inch below the bottom of the eyeball, at the bottom of the center of the bony orbit, high on the cheek. Tap firmly, but not hard enough to cause pain.
5. Tap the collarbone point five times again.
6. Take a second SUD rating and write it down. If it has decreased 2 or more points (which will be the case for most people), then continue with step 7 below. If there was no change, however, or if the change in the SUD was only 1 point, perform the correction for a psychological reversal, using the technique described in Chapter 4 (see page 84). Then repeat steps 1 through 6.

7. Perform the nine gamut treatments. Locate the gamut spot on the back of the hand, about an inch below the raised knuckles of the ring finger and little finger when making a fist. Begin tapping the gamut spot with two fingers of the opposite hand, about three to five times per second, and continue tapping while performing all nine steps below (tap five or six times for each of the nine gamut positions). It is very important to tap the gamut spot throughout all nine of these gamut treatments:

    - Open the eyes.
    - Close the eyes.
    - Open the eyes and point them down and to the left.
    - Point the eyes down and to the right.
    - Whirl the eyes around in a circle in one direction.
    - Whirl the eyes around in the opposite direction.
    - Hum a few bars of any tune aloud (more than a single note; rest the eyes).
    - Count aloud from one to five.
    - Hum the tune again.

8. Tap the collarbone point five times again.
9. Tap under the eye five times again.
10. Tap the collarbone point five times again.
11. Take still another SUD rating and write it down. If it has declined to 1 (which will happen with most people), move to step 12 below. But if it has decreased significantly yet is still not a 1, perform the mini PR correction as described

in Chapter 4 (see page 85), and repeat the treatment steps above.

12. To ensure that the improvements you've made are complete, perform the floor-to-ceiling eye roll (when the SUD is 2 or lower): Hold your head level and move your eyes down. Then begin tapping the gamut point as you move your eyes upward.

Obsession (OCD) Algorithm—Alternative 1

1. Tune the Thought Field—that is, intentionally think about the obsession that you are treating.
2. Using the Subjective Units of Distress (SUD) scale, rate the intensity of your urge to engage in the obsessive behavior at this moment. On this scale, 10 is the worst you could possibly feel, and 1 indicates absolutely no trace of upset. Write down the SUD rating.
3. Tap solidly five times under the arm, about four inches directly below the armpit, using rigid fingers. In men, this spot is under the arm about even with the nipple. Women can locate this spot by tapping at about the center of the bra under the arm.
4. Tap five times under the eye, about an inch below the bottom of the eyeball, at the bottom of the center of the bony orbit, high on the cheek. Tap firmly, but not hard enough to cause pain.
5. Tap the "collarbone point." To locate it, take two fingers of either hand and run them down the center of the throat to the top of the center collarbone notch. This is approximately even with the spot where a man would knot

his tie. From there, move straight down an additional inch. Then move to the right one inch. Tap this point five times.

6. Take a second SUD rating and write it down. If it has decreased 2 or more points (which will be the case for most people), then continue with step 7 below. If there was no change, however, or if the change in the SUD was only 1 point, perform the correction for a psychological reversal, using the technique described in Chapter 4 (see page 84). Then repeat steps 1 through 6.

7. Perform the nine gamut treatments. Locate the gamut spot on the back of the hand, about an inch below the raised knuckles of the ring finger and little finger when making a fist. Begin tapping the gamut spot with two fingers of the opposite hand, about three to five times per second, and continue tapping while performing all nine steps below (tap five or six times for each of the nine gamut positions). It is very important to tap the gamut spot throughout all nine of these gamut treatments:

    - Open the eyes.
    - Close the eyes.
    - Open the eyes and point them down and to the left.
    - Point the eyes down and to the right.
    - Whirl the eyes around in a circle in one direction.
    - Whirl the eyes around in the opposite direction.
    - Hum a few bars of any tune aloud (more than a single note; rest the eyes).
    - Count aloud from one to five.
    - Hum the tune again.

8. Tap solidly five times under the arm again.

9. Tap under the eye five times again.

10. Tap the collarbone point five times again.

11. Take still another SUD rating and write it down. If it has declined to 1 (which will happen with most people), move to step 12 below. But if it has decreased significantly yet is still not a 1, perform the mini PR correction as described in Chapter 4 (see page 85), and then repeat the treatment steps above.

12. To ensure that the improvements you've made are complete, perform the floor-to-ceiling eye roll (when the SUD is 2 or lower): Hold your head level and move your eyes down. Then begin tapping the gamut point as you move your eyes upward.

Obsession (OCD) Algorithm—Alternative 2

1. Tune the Thought Field—that is, intentionally think about the obsession that you are treating.

2. Using the Subjective Units of Distress (SUD) scale, rate the intensity of your urge to engage in the obsessive behavior at this moment. On this scale, 10 is the worst you could possibly feel, and 1 indicates absolutely no trace of upset. Write down the SUD rating.

3. Tap five times under the eye, about an inch below the bottom of the eyeball, at the bottom of the center of the bony orbit, high on the cheek. Tap firmly, but not hard enough to cause pain.

4. Tap solidly five times under the arm, about four inches directly below the armpit, using rigid fingers. In men, this

spot is under the arm about even with the nipple. Women can locate this spot by tapping at about the center of the bra under the arm.

5. Tap the "collarbone point." To locate it, take two fingers of either hand and run them down the center of the throat to the top of the center collarbone notch. This is approximately even with the spot where a man would knot his tie. From there, move straight down an additional inch. Then move to the right one inch. Tap this point five times.

6. Take a second SUD rating and write it down. If it has decreased 2 or more points (which will be the case for most people), then continue with step 7 below. If there was no change, however, or if the change in the SUD was only 1 point, perform the correction for a psychological reversal, using the technique described in Chapter 4 (see page 84). Then repeat steps 1 through 6.

7. Perform the nine gamut treatments. Locate the gamut spot on the back of the hand, about an inch below the raised knuckles of the ring finger and little finger when making a fist. Begin tapping the gamut spot with two fingers of the opposite hand, about three to five times per second, and continue tapping while performing all nine steps below (tap five or six times for each of the nine gamut positions). It is very important to tap the gamut spot throughout all nine of these gamut treatments:

   - Open the eyes.
   - Close the eyes.
   - Open the eyes and point them down and to the left.
   - Point the eyes down and to the right.
   - Whirl the eyes around in a circle in one direction.

- Whirl the eyes around in the opposite direction.
- Hum a few bars of any tune aloud (more than a single note; rest the eyes).
- Count aloud from one to five.
- Hum the tune again.

8. Tap under the eye five times again.
9. Tap solidly five times under the arm again.
10. Tap the collarbone point five times again.
11. Take still another SUD rating and write it down. If it has declined to 1 (which will happen with most people), move to step 12 below. But if it has decreased significantly, yet is still not a 1, perform the mini PR correction as described in Chapter 4 (see page 85), and then repeat the treatment steps above.
12. To ensure that the improvements you've made are complete, perform the floor-to-ceiling eye roll (when the SUD is 2 or lower): Hold your head level and move your eyes down. Then begin tapping the gamut point as you move your eyes upward.

GUILT

Many people have difficulty letting go of guilt. They may feel guilty about past behaviors or violations of personal commitments. Or their guilt may be related to the shirking of responsibilities or to extramarital affairs. Perhaps you can make a list of your own past regrets over which you still carry some heavy emotional baggage.

Guilt can be a disabling emotion, often related to events from decades earlier that can't be changed. But guilt can be eliminated with the following algorithm.

Guilt Algorithm

1. Tune the Thought Field—that is, intentionally think about the guilt that produces such emotional distress in your life.
2. Rate the intensity of your guilt at this moment, using the Subjective Units of Distress (SUD) scale. On this scale, 10 is the worst you could possibly feel, and 1 indicates absolutely no trace of upset. Write down the SUD rating.
3. Tap the "index finger spot" five times. It is located on the tip of the index (pointing) finger, on the side of that finger next to the thumb.
4. Tap the "collarbone point." To locate it, take two fingers of either hand and run them down the center of the throat to the top of the center collarbone notch. This is approximately even with the spot where a man would knot his tie. From there, move straight down an additional inch. Then move to the right one inch. Tap this point five times.
5. Take a second SUD rating and write it down. If it has decreased 2 or more points (which will be the case for most people), then continue with step 6 below. If there was no change, however, or if the change in the SUD was only 1 point, perform the correction for a psychological reversal, using the technique described in Chapter 4 (see page 84). Then repeat steps 1 through 5.

6. Perform the nine gamut treatments. Locate the gamut spot on the back of the hand, about an inch below the raised knuckles of the ring finger and little finger when making a fist. Begin tapping the gamut spot with two fingers of the opposite hand, about three to five times per second, and continue tapping while performing all nine steps below (tap five or six times for each of the nine gamut positions). It is very important to tap the gamut spot throughout all nine of these gamut treatments:
   - Open the eyes.
   - Close the eyes.
   - Open the eyes and point them down and to the left.
   - Point the eyes down and to the right.
   - Whirl the eyes around in a circle in one direction.
   - Whirl the eyes around in the opposite direction.
   - Hum a few bars of any tune aloud (more than a single note; rest the eyes).
   - Count aloud from one to five.
   - Hum the tune again.
7. Tap the index finger spot five times again.
8. Tap the collarbone point five times again.
9. Take still another SUD rating and write it down. If it has declined to 1 (which will happen with most people), move to step 10 below. But if it has decreased significantly yet is still not a 1, perform the mini PR correction as described in Chapter 4 (see page 85), and then repeat the treatment steps above.

10. To ensure that the improvements you've made are complete, perform the floor-to-ceiling eye roll (when the SUD is 2 or lower): Hold your head level and move your eyes down. Then begin tapping the gamut point as you move your eyes upward.

SHAME/EMBARRASSMENT

If you feel shame or embarrassment over events in your past or present, and if it is making it difficult for you to function in your day-to-day activities without emotional distress, then you should use the appropriate Thought Field Therapy algorithm. Within minutes, it can put feelings such as these behind you so you can lead your life without the disruption of unproductive emotions.

There are separate algorithms for shame and embarrassment. They are brief and can be carried out in just seconds.

Shame Algorithm

1. Tune the Thought Field—that is, intentionally think about the shame that you'd like to resolve.

2. Using the Subjective Units of Distress (SUD) scale, rate the degree of shame you feel at this moment when thinking of the incident associated with it. On this scale, 10 is the worst you could possibly feel, and 1 indicates absolutely no trace of shame. Write down the SUD rating.

3. Tap a treatment point on the center of the chin, just below the lip. Tap this point five times.

4. Take another SUD rating and write it down. If it has declined all the way to 1, move to step 5 below. But if it has

decreased significantly yet is still not a 1, perform the mini PR correction as described in Chapter 4 (see page 85), and then repeat the treatment steps above.

5. To ensure that the improvements you've made are complete, perform the floor-to-ceiling eye roll (when the SUD is 2 or lower): Hold your head level and move your eyes down. Then begin tapping the gamut point as you move your eyes upward.

Embarrassment Algorithm

1. Tune the Thought Field—that is, intentionally think about the embarrassment that you'd like to resolve.
2. Using the Subjective Units of Distress (SUD) scale, rate the degree of embarrassment you feel at this moment when thinking about the incident associated with it. On this scale, 10 is the worst you could possibly feel, and 1 indicates absolutely no trace of embarrassment. Write down the SUD rating.
3. Tap a treatment point on the upper lip below the nose. Tap this point five times.
4. Take another SUD rating and write it down. If it has declined all the way to 1, move to step 5 below. But if it has decreased significantly, but is still not a 1, perform the mini PR correction as described in Chapter 4 (see page 85), and then repeat the treatment steps above.
5. To ensure that the improvements you've made are complete, perform the floor-to-ceiling eye roll (when the SUD is 2 or lower): Hold your head level and move your eyes down. Then begin tapping the gamut point as you move your eyes upward.

JET LAG

Whether you're traveling across time zones for business or vacation, jet lag can leave you feeling fatigued and run-down. When your biological clock is disrupted, friends might suggest all kinds of stopgap measures to ease the symptoms, ranging from changes in diet to shifting your sleep/wake cycle several days before departure. But rarely do these eliminate the problem.

Most experts believe that jet lag is caused by changes in the traveler's eating and sleeping schedules. I can confirm the difficulty I once had constantly changing eating and sleeping patterns when I was a student and also worked on the graveyard shift at an automobile plant in Detroit. But I think there's more to jet lag than radical disruptions of the circadian rhythms. The earth's electromagnetic environment affects all living things, and I believe that the primary cause of jet lag is the rapid crossing of the north-south electromagnetic lines of force surrounding the earth as we travel in an easterly or westerly direction.

Traveling in an eastward direction had always been particularly difficult for me (others find westward travel more difficult). In the past, I would need several days—sometimes as much as a full week—of adjustment when jetting to Europe, no matter what strategies I tried. But since I've been using the Thought Field Therapy algorithm below, I have been able to eliminate all traces of jet lag in minutes. As you'll see, there are separate algorithms for traveling from west to east, and from east to west.

Four important points:

- Perform the algorithm every waking hour during your flight. If you plan to nap on the plane, do the treatment before going to sleep and after awakening. If you've slept during most or all of the flight, perform the algorithm after your arrival to minimize jet lag; you can also repeat the "recipe" again and again at your destination if you should ever feel symptoms.

- If you're performing the algorithms on the flight itself, you won't be feeling any symptoms of jet lag yet, so you won't be able to determine an SUD rating at that time. However, when you're using the algorithms at your destination, and you're feeling symptoms associated with the travel, then you can arrive at SUD ratings during the algorithms to evaluate how well the treatments are working.
- Although the algorithms are effective for the vast majority of people, if they don't work for you, reverse them—that is, perform the east to west algorithm when traveling west to east, and vice versa.
- If you're particularly susceptible to jet lag problems, avoid consuming alcohol during the flight. Airline cabins are pressurized at an altitude comparable to about 8,000 feet, which can complicate adaptation problems for some people who drink.

Jet Lag Algorithm—West to East

1. Tune the Thought Field—that is, intentionally think about the jet lag that produces such upset in your life. (If you are performing this algorithm while in flight, and thus not yet experiencing jet lag symptoms, simply turn your attention to the rapid travel you're doing.)
2. Rate your distress level at this moment, using the Subjective Units of Distress (SUD) scale. On this scale, 10 is the worst you could possibly feel, and 1 indicates absolutely no trace of upset. Write down the SUD rating.
3. Tap five times under the eye, about an inch below the bottom of the eyeball, at the bottom of the center of the bony orbit, high on the cheek. Tap firmly, but not hard enough to cause pain.

4. Tap the "collarbone point." To locate it, take two fingers of either hand and run them down the center of the throat to the top of the center collarbone notch. This is approximately even with the spot where a man would knot his tie. From there, move straight down an additional inch. Then move to the right one inch. Tap this point five times.

5. Take a second SUD rating and write it down. If it has decreased 2 or more points (which will be the case for most people), then continue with step 6 below. If there was no change, however, or if the change in the SUD was only 1 point, perform the correction for a psychological reversal, using the technique described in Chapter 4 (see page 84). Then repeat steps 1 through 5.

6. Perform the nine gamut treatments. Locate the gamut spot on the back of the hand, about an inch below the raised knuckles of the ring finger and little finger when making a fist. Begin tapping the gamut spot with two fingers of the opposite hand, about three to five times per second, and continue tapping while performing all nine steps below (tap five or six times for each of the nine gamut positions). It is very important to tap the gamut spot throughout all nine of these gamut treatments:

   - Open the eyes.
   - Close the eyes.
   - Open the eyes and point them down and to the left.
   - Point the eyes down and to the right.
   - Whirl the eyes around in a circle in one direction.
   - Whirl the eyes around in the opposite direction.
   - Hum a few bars of any tune aloud (more than a single note; rest the eyes).

- Count aloud from one to five.
- Hum the tune again.

7. Tap under the eye five times again.
8. Tap the collarbone point five times again.
9. Take still another SUD rating and write it down. If it has declined to 1 (which will happen with most people), move to step 10 below. But if it has decreased significantly yet is still not a 1, perform the mini PR correction as described in Chapter 4 (see page 85), and then repeat the treatment steps above.
10. To ensure that the improvements you've made are complete, perform the floor-to-ceiling eye roll (when the SUD is 2 or lower): Hold your head level and move your eyes down. Then begin tapping the gamut point as you move your eyes upward.

Jet Lag Algorithm—East to West

1. Tune the Thought Field—that is, intentionally think about the jet lag that produces such upset in your life. (If you are performing this algorithm while in flight, and thus not yet experiencing jet lag symptoms, simply turn your attention to the rapid travel you're doing.)
2. Rate your distress level at this moment, using the Subjective Units of Distress (SUD) scale. On this scale, 10 is the worst you could possibly feel, and 1 indicates absolutely no trace of upset. Write down the SUD rating.
3. Tap solidly five times under the arm, about four inches directly below the armpit, using rigid fingers. In men, this spot is under the arm about even with the nipple. Women

can locate this spot by tapping at about the center of the bra under the arm.

4. Tap the "collarbone point." To locate it, take two fingers of either hand and run them down the center of the throat to the top of the center collarbone notch. This is approximately even with the spot where a man would knot his tie. From there, move straight down an additional inch. Then move to the right one inch. Tap this point five times.

5. Take a second SUD rating and write it down. If it has decreased 2 or more points (which will be the case for most people), then continue with step 6 below. If there was no change, however, or if the change in the SUD was only 1 point, perform the correction for a psychological reversal, using the technique described in Chapter 4 (see page 84). Then repeat steps 1 through 5.

6. Perform the nine gamut treatments. Locate the gamut spot on the back of the hand, about an inch below the raised knuckles of the ring finger and little finger when making a fist. Begin tapping the gamut spot with two fingers of the opposite hand, about three to five times per second, and continue tapping while performing all nine steps below (tap five or six times for each of the nine gamut positions). It is important to tap the gamut spot throughout all nine of these gamut treatments:

   - Open the eyes.
   - Close the eyes.
   - Open the eyes and point them down and to the left.
   - Point the eyes down and to the right.
   - Whirl the eyes around in a circle in one direction.
   - Whirl the eyes around in the opposite direction.

- Hum a few bars of any tune aloud (more than a single note; rest the eyes).
- Count aloud from one to five.
- Hum the tune again.

7. Tap under the arm five times again.
8. Tap the collarbone point five times again.
9. Take still another SUD rating and write it down. If it has declined to 1 (which will happen with most people), move to step 10 below. But if it has decreased significantly yet is still not a 1, perform the mini PR correction as described in Chapter 4 (see page 85), and then repeat the treatment steps above.
10. To ensure that the improvements you've made are complete, perform the floor-to-ceiling eye roll (when the SUD is 2 or lower): Hold your head level and move your eyes down. Then begin tapping the gamut point as you move your eyes upward.

PHYSICAL PAIN

Millions of people live with physical pain every day of their lives. They have splitting and stabbing headaches. Or their neck is hot and burning. Their back is sore and stinging. Their knee is throbbing.

Physical pain can crush the body and spirit, and at its worst, it can destroy any semblance of a normal life. In desperation, people become addicted to painkilling drugs or submit to nerve blocks or risky surgery, often with little to show for it at the end of the day except the same excruciating pain they began with. Just as main-stream psychotherapy has a weak track record in healing emotional pain, traditional medicine fares poorly in permanently resolving headaches, back pain, and even the pain of metastisized cancer.

But Thought Field Therapy can help. The physical pain algorithm works for the majority of people, and does so rapidly and safely. I have seen it ease or eliminate headaches, back pain, and many other types of discomfort.

Physical Pain Algorithm

1. Tune the Thought Field—that is, intentionally think about the physical pain you're experiencing.
2. Rate your pain level at the moment, using the Subjective Units of Distress (SUD) scale, with 10 representing the most intense pain possible, and 1 indicating absolutely no trace of pain. Write down the SUD rating.
3. Locate the gamut spot on the back of the hand, about an inch below the raised knuckles of the ring finger and little finger when making a fist. Tap this gamut spot fifty times, using two fingers of the opposite hand.
4. Tap the "collarbone point." To locate it, take two fingers of either hand and run them down the center of the throat to the top of the center collarbone notch. This is approximately even with the spot where a man would knot his tie. From there, move straight down an additional inch. Then move to the right one inch. Tap this point five times.
5. Take a second SUD rating and write it down. If it has decreased 2 or more points (which will be the case for most people), then continue with step 6 below. If there was no change, however, or if the change in the SUD was only 1 point, perform the correction for a psychological reversal,

using the technique described in Chapter 4 (see page 84). Then repeat steps 1 through 5.

6. Perform the nine gamut treatments. Locate the gamut spot on the back of the hand (see step 3 above). Then begin tapping the gamut spot with two fingers of the opposite hand, about three to five times per second, and continue tapping while performing all nine steps below (tap five or six times for each of the nine gamut positions). It is very important to tap the gamut spot throughout all nine of these gamut treatments:

   - Open the eyes.
   - Close the eyes.
   - Open the eyes and point them down and to the left.
   - Point the eyes down and to the right.
   - Whirl the eyes around in a circle in one direction.
   - Whirl the eyes around in the opposite direction.
   - Hum a few bars of any tune aloud (more than a single note; rest the eyes).
   - Count aloud from one to five.
   - Hum the tune again.

7. Tap the gamut spot fifty times again.

8. Tap the collarbone point five times again.

9. Take still another SUD rating and write it down. If it has declined to 1 (which will happen with most people), move to step 10 below. But if it has decreased significantly yet is still not a 1, perform the mini PR correction as described

in Chapter 4 (see page 85), and then repeat the treatment steps above.

10. To ensure that the improvements you've made are complete, perform the floor-to-ceiling eye roll (when the SUD is 2 or lower): Hold your head level and move your eyes down. Then begin tapping the gamut point as you move your eyes upward.

6

TIPS FOR TROUBLESHOOTING

BY NOW, I HOPE you've tried the Thought Field Therapy algorithm for your particular problem, whether it is anxiety, trauma, a phobia, a panic disorder, or depression. If you're like most people, after using the algorithm just once, your problem has been completely eliminated, or at least you've experienced a dramatic improvement in your well-being. Even if you've been trying to treat a physical disorder—perhaps a pain problem—you should be feeling better after just a few minutes of TFT.

One of my colleagues recently described his experience treating a twenty-four-year-old woman I'll call Cynthia. She was a receptionist for a medical practice, and she would have severe anxiety and panic attacks when patients would come into the office feeling nauseous, or even when they would merely describe their nausea and vomiting over the phone to her. Cynthia's anxiety, which caused spells of crying and unusual sweating, was interfering terribly with her job and her life. At times, when patients called for appointments and described having vomiting symptoms, she would tell them to see another doctor. She just couldn't deal with it. Finally, she asked for a transfer to the office's medical records department so she wouldn't be confronted with ill patients.

Cynthia recognized that she needed some help and chose Thought Field Therapy. As her treatment began, she was asked to think about her problem (tune the Thought Field), and she got in touch with the intensity of her panic and anxiety. She evaluated her SUD on a 10-point scale and rated it "ten-plus." Then she was guided through the TFT treatment. It took just minutes. When it was over, she evaluated her SUD again. It had declined to a 1! She was challenged to try hard to become upset thinking about the problem, but she could not get even a little anxious. She broke into a smile and then began laughing. She felt she had been cured.

Cynthia went back to her receptionist's job, and she has had no problems interacting with patients suffering from nausea. She freely talks with friends and family without any concerns that the subjects of nausea and vomiting will come up. And by the way, not long after her TFT treatment, Cynthia became pregnant, and she had no morning sickness—nor was she the slightest bit worried about experiencing those kinds of symptoms.

HOW LONG WILL IT LAST?

Nearly everyone treated with Thought Field Therapy is delighted with the results. If you're like most people, you should experience significant improvements in or, more often, a complete elimination of your problem. When evaluating the SUD rating immediately after the treatment, some individuals have trouble even assigning a number to it. This almost always indicates a SUD of 1.

My clients and other psychotherapists often ask me how long the treatment benefits will last. Whenever I hear this question, I am intrigued. After all, in the pre-TFT days when I was practicing traditional psychotherapy, no one ever asked how long treatment improvements would persist. There was a good reason for this: in most cases, *no improvement occurred*, and thus there was nothing of substance *to* last!

Because TFT is so unconventional and produces results so rapidly, some patients are initially convinced that improvements can't persist. But Thought Field Therapy is *not* a short-term fix. Mary, my first patient, was cured of her water phobia after a single treatment, and that cure has endured for nearly two decades, without a trace of her phobia ever arising again! Her frequent and terrifying nightmares, which had been related to the phobia, had become a defining part of her life, but they disappeared after TFT and have *never* recurred!

The quick and lasting effects of TFT are not only important to you, the client, but also to therapists who work with this technique. One of my colleagues, therapist Monica Pignotti, recently wrote an article in the newsletter *The Thought Field* in which she cited the high incidence of burnout among mainstream therapists by the time they reach middle age. But she emphasized that this same kind of burnout is not seen with TFT practitioners. "In my opinion," she wrote, "this burnout phenomenon comes from therapists who truly want to help people—having to sit with clients for session after session, watching them suffer, struggling valiantly to help them, but not having the skill or knowledge to produce any kind of clinically significant changes." In contrast, she said, practitioners trained in TFT are able to help people rapidly and permanently, which is exciting and fulfilling.

Can you expect the same? If TFT collapsed all of the perturbations, the problem shouldn't return. That's what happens with the overwhelming majority of people. But if the emotional turmoil doesn't disappear completely after TFT, or if it returns after a period of time, there are corrective actions you can take to move toward complete healing.

THE MOST COMMON PROBLEMS

If you didn't achieve the results you wanted from your first use of TFT, here are some factors to keep in mind:

- Some cases may require more than one TFT treatment. The first time you use an algorithm, it might not get rid of all of the perturbations. When this happens, parts of the Thought Field may not have been tuned properly, and thus the perturbations weren't treated effectively in the first attempt. What's the solution? A few people may benefit from repeating the algorithm—in some cases, up to five times on different occasions to achieve maximum results. Fortunately, the algorithms are easy to do again. In fact, you'll become more comfortable using them each succeeding time. After one or more additional treatments, any remaining perturbations can usually be eradicated. With patience, most people lower their SUD score to 1.

- On rare occasions, people have trouble performing the algorithm from beginning to end. The portion that seems to be the most difficult for a very small number of individuals involves the eye movements—specifically, the positioning or rolling of the eyes that is part of the gamut series. About one in a thousand people finds that moving his or her eyes causes dizziness or anxiety. There's certainly no health danger associated with this, but it's not a particularly comfortable feeling, either. If it happens to you, here's my suggestion: simply *imagine* performing the eye movements while tapping the gamut spot. This can be just as effective as actually doing them. Also, if you wear contact lenses, proceed through these eye movements with care to keep from dislodging the contacts or hurting your eyes.

- Occasionally, when individuals have suppressed their psychological distress (for example, they've suppressed a traumatic event or a fear of public speaking), they may not even be able to get a SUD reading for their condition. While they know that a problem exists, the SUD is a 1 when they think about it. Even in this case, however, the appropriate TFT algorithm can successfully treat the problem.

Interestingly, when one of my colleagues was unable to get a SUD reading related to a traumatic event that had occurred in her own life many years earlier, a Heart Rate Variability test showed—much to her surprise—that significant autonomic nervous system imbalances occurred when she turned her attention to the trauma. She treated the distress with Thought Field Therapy, and follow-up HRV readings indicated a powerful improvement. Were it not for the HRV test, she might not have thought that the trauma had been affecting her at all—and that it could be resolved with TFT.

So remember, even if you aren't able to get a SUD reading, treat the problem anyway. Real healing will take place with TFT.

• Another phenomenon that occurs occasionally is a delayed treatment response, or as I call it, "inertial delay." Although rare, there may be an unanticipated gap between the TFT treatment and its perceived benefits. In these cases, no perturbations have been left untreated, but still the positive effects don't occur immediately.

I recall treating a young man who was in terrible emotional distress over the loss of a love. After TFT, he found that his SUD level had decreased somewhat, but the agony lingered. Then, a few minutes later, even though there had been no additional treatment, his distress completely vanished.

Sometimes this delay lasts minutes; other times, it may continue for hours or, rarely, even a day or more. Then the positive effects of TFT finally take place quite dramatically.

What's the reason for this inertial delay? When it happens, toxins are often present (I'll talk more about toxins later). These delays are also more likely to occur in older individuals.

ARE YOU A COMPLEX CASE?

In traditional psychotherapy, patients may be in treatment for years and still never achieve the results they're seeking. In TFT, however, problems are usually eliminated in minutes. If they aren't, the case may be "complex." Certain psychological conditions, such as agoraphobia and severe addictions, tend to be more complex than others. Some people may have multiple problems that need to be treated layer by layer.

To illustrate this latter situation, which I call the "tooth, shoe, lump" principle, let me relate the following fictional story:

A man develops a miserable, throbbing toothache. He calls his dentist's office and is told to come over at once. "There are no openings in the schedule," the receptionist tells him, "but we'll squeeze you in as soon as we can."

Rushing to leave for the dentist's office, the man puts on the first pair of shoes he comes across, overlooking the fact that the shoes are pinching his toes. Because his tooth pain is so severe, he doesn't even notice how irritating the shoes are.

When the man arrives at the dentist's office, he takes a seat in the waiting room, perching himself directly on a very uncomfortable lump in the sofa. But again, he doesn't even notice it because his tooth hurts so much.

Within minutes, the dentist enters the waiting room and tells the man that he won't be able to treat him for another ninety minutes. But, noticing the patient's pain, the dentist offers to give him a shot of Novocain to temporarily relieve the discomfort.

Within minutes, the man's toothache has subsided. As it does, he suddenly becomes aware that his feet are in terrible pain. He looks down and sees that he has put on an old, poorly fitting pair of shoes. He unties their laces and slips out of them. As he does, his feet feel much better. At that moment, however, his attention suddenly turns to that uncomfortable lump in the sofa that he has been sitting on. He quickly gets up and moves to a nearby chair in the waiting room. At last he is pain-free.

For some people whose cases are complex, their treatment often unfolds in a way similar to the man in the dentist's waiting room. They may have a hierarchy of problems—not just depression, for example, but also anxiety and perhaps the aftereffects of a traumatic event. Before and during TFT, they may have difficulty discriminating between one problem and another. All they know is that they feel bad. So while the initial treatment may eliminate one area of distress, they may still feel terrible because their other disorders remain. It may take some sophisticated diagnostic and treatment procedures to eradicate all of their problems and set them on the road to complete healing. I'll talk more about this later.

THE PERILS OF PSYCHOLOGICAL REVERSAL

Sometimes individuals are treated with Thought Field Therapy and they don't get much better. Even though the algorithms are carried out exactly as instructed, they still haven't experienced healing. Of course, this would cause plenty of frustration—were it not for the ability to discover what's causing this roadblock to healing.

If you're having trouble getting to 1 on the SUD scale, psychological reversal is likely the cause. As you may recall from Chapter 4, psychological reversal, or PR, is actually the most common impediment to recovery in TFT or any other usually successful treatment. It is a state or condition of being that interferes with healing and keeps TFT (or any other treatment) from working.

At one time or another, all of us are in a state of psychological reversal. If a PR is present, you won't be able to collapse the existing perturbations and effectively eliminate the problem you're trying to treat. This PR appears related to a blockage or a polarity reversal of the energy flow within the body. Fortunately, PRs are correctable, usually within seconds. In fact, were it not for the correction of this psychological reversal, the success rate associated with TFT would be about 40 percent lower than it is.

There are often some obvious clues that a PR is present. For example, although we really don't know exactly why, people with PR frequently reverse the order of letters or numbers; if they are told a phone number of 434-1632, they may write down or dial 434-3216 (a special proofreader's mark exists for this type of mistake, which is an indication of how common it is). They might also confuse directional concepts—saying "up" when they mean "down," or "left" when they mean "right." (Interestingly, while they may say "south" when they mean "north," they will not say "east" or "west" when they mean "south.") They may reverse certain actions—for example, placing a cooked casserole in the oven rather than the refrigerator, or vice versa—or reverse colors as they describe them in a color chart. A PR may also contribute to a negative attitude, or a bad or destructive mood, and it can impair everyday performance and productivity. While the severity and intensity of a PR may vary, it can and must be corrected before TFT (or any effective therapy) can have a positive impact.

Psychological reversal is found not only in psychological disorders, but it can also be present in people with chronic physical illnesses, including cancer. A study at New York University years ago found that 96 percent of cancer patients had a polarity reversal (or "negative polarity") as measured by sensitive instruments, compared to only 5 percent of patients without cancerous tumors. (Much more research needs to be done in this area, but it's possible that just as psychological problems cannot be successfully treated if a PR is present, something similar may also interfere with the treatment of some cancer cases.) It may be that correcting the PR can free the body to respond to treatments that would otherwise be effective.

Eliminating Psychological Reversal

If you have signs or symptoms suggestive of psychological reversal, or if the healing of a particular problem seems blocked, you may need to administer a PR-specific correction.

In Chapter 4, I described the technique for correcting a PR; to repeat, it involves two steps:

1. Find the "PR spot" on the outer edge of either hand, about midway between the wrist and the base of the little finger.
2. Using two fingers of the other hand, tap the PR spot five times.

Once PR has been successfully corrected—which takes only a few seconds—then the TFT treatment can be resumed. At this point, TFT can rapidly resolve the underlying problem you're trying to treat.

Sometimes, the PR correction itself is all that needs to be done. I recall one case involving a beautiful young girl, nearly four years old, who had spent a long day on a boat with her parents and some other relatives. Suddenly, this little girl (I'll call her Judy) began crying, screaming, and kicking without explanation. All of the adults nearby tried to calm her down, but to no avail. Because Judy was in such agony, the people around her were suffering as well.

Judy's misery persisted for an hour. Finally, her mother turned to me and asked, "Is there anything you can do?" I suggested the PR treatment. Her mother felt there was nothing to lose, and as I guided her, she gently but firmly tapped on the side of her daughter's hand.

Quite literally in a matter of seconds, Judy was transformed. This little girl, who had been hysterical one moment, instantly stopped crying. She calmly looked at the people around her and at her surroundings. Within seconds, she began interacting with these adults as if nothing had happened.

A number of years ago, I was the guest on Tom Snyder's television talk show, and I had the opportunity to demonstrate a psychological reversal correction on live TV. Snyder had an intense fear of heights, and we agreed that he would try to climb a ladder after I treated him with TFT's phobia algorithm. Though the algorithm works for most people, it did nothing for Snyder. So I administered the brief PR correction and then repeated the algorithm. After this simple correction, all traces of his fear were gone. He climbed the ladder without hesitation or anxiety.

Psychological reversal is something traditional psychotherapists never consider; in fact, they aren't even aware of it. There are many reasons why their success rates are so low, and PR certainly contributes to it. But PR treatment can be repeated as often as needed, to put you back on track for healing.

Remember, if TFT has ended your desire for a cigarette, or eliminated the emotional despair you felt over the loss of a love, but then those feelings return, a PR has probably surfaced. Until it is corrected, that reversal will be an absolute block to permanent recovery. Whether you're trying to lose weight, stop smoking, or conquer a social phobia, you won't reach your goal if a PR is present.

Putting PR Correction to the Test

Dr. Robert Blaich, a leading practitioner in applied kinesiology, has conducted research evaluating approaches for improving human performance. One of those studies involved individuals who were already highly successful, but who sought ways of further enhancing their achievements. Dr. Blaich compared a number of techniques, including PR correction, measuring their effects on performance by evaluating changes in the reading and comprehension skills of these volunteers. The study concluded that the simple correction of psychological reversal was the most effective therapy of all those tested, including many complex treatments, and produced the greatest possible changes. Dr. Blaich also told me that PR correction turned out to be the most valuable tool for helping elite athletes maximize their performance and break records set by themselves and others.

In Chapter 3, I described another TFT study involving the use of Thought Field Therapy in callers to radio talk shows. About 30 percent of the individuals who participated in the study did not receive immediate relief from their problem, and I felt that they were psychologically reversed. To confirm the presence of a PR, I guided each of these callers through the PR correction procedure, but without really explaining to them what I was doing. After this treatment, we repeated the TFT algorithm. Twenty of the twenty-two reversed callers responded immediately when the algorithm was repeated. (The two exceptions had a more complex type of reversal that, at the time, couldn't be corrected immediately.)

I can't overemphasize the importance of correcting for psychological reversal. Discovering the existence of a PR and an effective treatment for it has allowed me to achieve an unprecedented rate of success in resolving psychological problems that have resisted all other forms of therapy. As powerful as TFT is, it would be less effective—with success rates perhaps 40 to 50 percent lower—were it not for the ability to recognize and correct psychological reversal.

Remember, whether you're trying to cure a phobia, depression, an eating disorder, or panic attacks, Thought Field Therapy cannot succeed when you are in a state of psychological reversal. Jack Paar once said, "Did you ever feel that life is an obstacle course and you are the biggest obstacle?" Thanks to PR correction, such people can rapidly change this pattern and also eliminate the barriers to their own healing.

ARE TOXINS WEIGHING YOU DOWN?

Here's a scenario that sometimes occurs: You put the TFT algorithms to work, and within minutes, a problem that may have bothered you for years has been eliminated. But then you're faced with an undesirable turn of events, and quite unexpectedly, the problem returns.

In many cases, toxins are to blame. Even though the benefits of TFT will persist over time in the great majority of individuals, stress sometimes sabotages the treatment, typically in the form of an exogenous substance or toxin. Without knowing it, you may react to toxins in ways that can disrupt the balance of your body's energy system and cause recently eliminated problems to resurface. So if your problems return, you need to consider whether an external factor—exposure to an environmental toxin, consumption of a food to which you're sensitive, or the presence of an infection—is the cause. Smoking, for example, is a common toxin and will often undo a successful treatment. A complete cure can be undone by a factor like this, with the problem resurfacing as the toxin disrupts the homeostasis of the body.

Just how powerful can these toxins be? Years ago, before I had become aware of toxins, I was experiencing severe and chronic fatigue. I constantly felt run-down and achy. It was as though I had the flu all the time. More than a dozen physicians, chiropractors, and acupuncturists evaluated me, but none of them could find the cause or provide relief.

I recall seeing an experienced acupuncturist in his seventies, who had been trained in China, where his family had practiced acupuncture for generations. During our first meeting, he wasted no time in offering a simple explanation for my fatigue: "What do you expect?" he said. "You're getting old!" I seriously questioned whether my fatigue could simply be attributed to aging. After all, there were periods when I felt very energetic and I was just as old on those days as I was on days when I was exhausted (I was only fifty-six years old at the time). But the acupuncturist ignored what I said. He treated me with acupuncture needles in the arms and legs, and then sent me home with several herbs that he asked me to consume as teas. I was a compliant patient and followed his advice conscientiously.

Unfortunately, the herbs didn't make me feel better. In fact, they actually left me even more fatigued. I came to the conclusion that these herbs were toxic to my system—and just as significantly, that perhaps other toxins were responsible for the chronic fatigue that all the other doctors had been unable to treat.

I began making a series of discoveries that led me to recognize that I am a highly toxin-sensitive person. I identified a number of toxins that were undermining my health (they included wheat, vinegar, and cherries, among other foods). I also learned that toxins were actually interfering with my ability to cure my own fear of heights, which I was able to do with TFT once the toxins were eliminated (I had cured hundreds of others, but I had to make some new discoveries in order to cure my own fear of heights).

Since then, I've treated many patients whose well-being had been undermined by toxins. For example, there was a nineteen-year-old man I'll call Jeff. He had been in an automobile accident and in the aftermath couldn't drive a car without becoming panicky. Although TFT treated Jeff successfully for this panic disorder, it would return whenever he got into his car.

I suspected the presence of a toxin and learned that Jeff smoked cigarettes whenever he drove. Nicotine is a toxin that commonly sabotages the improvements already produced by a TFT algorithm. That's what happened with Jeff. Using Voice Technology (an advanced form of TFT), we diagnosed the source of his problem, and then with treatment eliminated smoking from his life for good. I treated him again with Thought Field Therapy, and as a result, his panic disorder has now been gone for more than two years.

Common Toxins

Some common substances seem unlikely toxins. For example, while cigarettes are an obvious source of toxicity (everyone now knows they're a poison), consuming wheat or corn is just as likely to cause problems in some people. Why do foods like these, which we generally think of as healthy, trigger toxic reactions in some individuals? The explanation lies in the chemicals in all plants, some of which are defensive agents to protect against external predators. Most people are able to consume these foods without any adverse reaction because their bodies manufacture enzymes that protect them from these poisons. For them, a food like wheat can be a very healthy part of their diet. But for individuals without those enzymes, wheat can ravage their bodies. (Interestingly, many people have toxic reactions to their favorite food.)

Keep in mind that toxins are different than allergies, which are immune system responses. The toxins I'm talking about are actual *poisons*. They won't kill you, but by disrupting your body's homeostasis, they may threaten your health. However, if you can identify and stay away from them for a period of time, your internal energy system will have an opportunity to heal, and you can keep your psychological and physical health problems in check. I have found that some people, after they've been toxin-free for two months, are able to have some of the problematic foods once every four days without adverse reactions.

Here are some common toxins:

- Wheat
- Corn

- Sugar
- Mayonnaise
- Vinegar
- Eggs
- Milk and other dairy products
- Coffee
- Tea
- Alcohol
- Tobacco
- Perfume
- Laundry soap
- Cleaning fluid
- Deodorizers
- Scented tissue
- Dyes
- Clothing materials (cotton, wool, etc.)
- Various chemicals (in clothing, carpets, upholstery, paint, etc.)
- Certain medications
- Pesticides

Upon ingestion or exposure to a toxic substance, most people exhibit one or more of the following symptoms:

- An increase in pulse rate
- Water retention

- Constipation or diarrhea
- Red ears or nose
- "Sticky" feces
- Weight gain
- Extreme tiredness

If you're skeptical that toxins like these are responsible for the psychological and physical problems in your life, ask a TFT practitioner to give you a Heart Rate Variability (HRV) test before and after exposure to toxins. For example, take the HRV test while wearing a garment known to be toxic, and then take it again after removing it. The HRV printout will clearly show the effect that toxins are having on the heart and the autonomic nervous system, which in turn reflect your overall well-being. Or consume a toxic substance and then remove it from your diet; your HRV readings will go from imbalanced to normal. By working with an authority trained in TFT's Voice Technology (I'll discuss Voice Technology in more detail later), you can identify the toxins that have undermined your treatment. Once you eliminate them from your diet or environment, you'll be back on the path to healing. A Voice Technology expert may even be able to recommend nutritional products that can help eliminate toxins from the body.

A Few Case Studies

Once a toxin is identified, it takes some care to ensure that you avoid exposure to it. I recall treating a Thought Field Therapy trainee I'll call Sandra. Sandra, in her early forties, had experienced an anxiety problem all of her life. Although I was able to eliminate it by treating her with TFT, it kept returning—a sure sign that a toxin is present. We identified this problematic substance as wheat, and I told Sandra to avoid it completely. I also instructed her to call me immediately if her anxiety resurfaced. "Be prepared to tell me what you ingested, and we'll find out why the anxiety returned," I told her.

Four days later, on a Sunday in the late afternoon, Sandra called. She said, "This is the longest time in thirty years that I've been free of anxiety, and I'm very grateful for that. But it came back today."

"Did you consume any wheat?"

"No. I know I'm not supposed to, so I'm being very careful to stay away from it."

I asked Sandra to tell me everything she had eaten that day. At one point, she said, "We went to the zoo in the afternoon, and I had an ice-cream cone."

We had found the culprit. "The cone! There's wheat in it!" I reminded her. It was the first step back to renewed healing. The treatment was repeated and her anxiety was eliminated.

Sometimes the detective work gets complex. A psychotherapist named Dan had suffered from depression for thirty years, and despite being in therapy most of that time and trying various antidepressant medications, nothing seemed to help him. With Thought Field Therapy, however, I eliminated his depression, and then I checked him for toxins (because his depression had persisted for so long, I strongly believed that toxins were an issue). Through Voice Technology, I discovered that corn was a toxin for him, and I asked him to remove it from his diet. As with Sandra, I also told him to call me if symptoms of depression resurfaced.

Sure enough, only three hours after I had treated him, Dan called. The depression was back.

"What have you eaten since we last spoke?"

"Nothing!" he responded matter-of-factly. "I haven't had *anything* to eat. I haven't had *anything* to drink."

I fired more questions at him. I asked him to recall in detail everything he had done in the previous three hours.

At one point, Dan said, "I wrote a couple letters."

That caught my attention. "Did you lick any stamps?"

"Sure."

"Well, there's corn syrup in the glue."

The corn had made his depression return.

Once toxins are eliminated, you can usually expect improvements almost instantly—but not always. One of my colleagues was treating a patient who had suffered from chronic pain for fifteen years. He had successfully lowered the client's SUD from a 10 to a 4, but it resisted going any lower. That's when I was called in to help.

Within minutes, we had identified and eliminated several toxins, but still the SUD wouldn't budge. Finally, I concluded that the client was experiencing "inertial delay" (see page 173). I suggested that he return home and assured him that he would likely notice some additional improvement soon, since no more perturbations were present.

Sure enough, he did. Four hours later, he phoned my colleague and was absolutely thrilled. "The pain is completely gone," he says. "I haven't felt this good in years!"

By the way, the concept of toxins is really nothing new. Many alternative doctors know about them, and I'm certainly not the first to recognize them. My particular discovery, however, is that toxins can disrupt or undo a cure, not only in psychotherapy, but in medicine, too.

THE ADVANCED THERAPIES

As I wrote in the opening pages of this book, the Thought Field Therapy algorithms work for 75 to 80 percent of people. That's a remarkable success record for the standard "recipes" that I've discovered and developed over many years. It is particularly extraordinary in a field where cures occur, at best, infrequently. Even so, if you're one of the 20 percent or so who aren't successful in reducing their SUD score to 1 with TFT, don't despair. My more recent discoveries have taken TFT to levels far more sophisticated than the algorithms, producing success rates that approach 100 percent! Even the toughest problems can be managed effectively with these advanced levels of TFT: Causal Diagnosis and Voice Technology. They are reserved for only the most difficult, complex cases.

To use these advanced levels of Thought Field Therapy, you will need the one-on-one guidance of a practitioner trained and experienced in "Callahan Techniques—TFT." They are not something you can do on your own. In the appendix of this book, I'll guide you in finding a specialist who can work with you, often over the phone (if toxins are believed to be a problem, he or she might also refer you to someone with advanced training in that area). As with the algorithms, these treatments are usually brief, involve tapping specific diagnosed points on the body, and very often require just one treatment session. (Note: A number of therapists who claim they do TFT have not been properly trained; use of the term *Callahan Techniques* ensures that a practitioner has received the necessary training.)

Although explaining these techniques in great detail is beyond the scope of this book, let me briefly introduce you to them.

Causal Diagnosis

When an algorithm is ineffective, Causal Diagnosis is the next step. It is a dynamic procedure that reveals the specific causal constituents (perturbations) that cause a particular psychological problem, in their correct order. It also identifies precisely which treatment should be used to eliminate the particular emotional distress. Causal diagnosis was used to discover the algorithms you'll find in this book.

Voice Technology

Voice Technology (VT) is the most sophisticated, accurate, and refined form of Thought Field Therapy now available. It can be used when neither algorithms nor Causal Diagnosis have produced healing, perhaps because remaining perturbations have not been detected and eliminated. VT relies solely on the voice for diagnosis and treatment selection. Like fingerprints, the voice has distinct characteristics that can be reliably analyzed. And because it involves only the voice, this entire process can be conducted on the phone.

VT is not influenced by language, inflection, or content. Nor does telephone transmission, which removes much of the information in the voice for efficiency, interfere with the process of detecting and decoding perturbations. The patient tunes the Thought Field, and then the relevant perturbation(s) can be identified.

When using VT, the number of points tapped is often much higher than with the algorithms because the problem is more complex and due to many more perturbations. There are twelve major points associated with the algorithms, although only about nine are typically used; with VT, however, hundreds of tapped points (including many that are used repeatedly) are sometimes needed, and as with the algorithms, they must be tapped in a particular sequence.

VT is extremely powerful, producing an extraordinarily high cure rate that approaches perfection. New discoveries just in the last two years have taken VT to an unprecedented success level of 97 to 99 percent! This rate of healing has been reported by one VT clinician after another, indicating the replicable nature and surprising power of this cutting-edge therapy.

Success Stories

One of my colleagues, a psychotherapist I'll call Denny, had experienced migraine headaches for years. He had tried many types of mainstream and alternative treatments but found no relief. In a typical week, he had migraines six of every seven days. He was spending $800 a month, sometimes more, on injections of a drug called Imitrex in an attempt to bring his headaches under control. But although this powerful drug provided short-term pain relief, it was not a cure, nor did it prevent future attacks. His level of frustration—and pain—was extremely high.

Denny was treated with Voice Technology, and the results were remarkable (he later went through VT training to learn how to administer this advanced form of therapy in his own practice). After a single treatment, he was able to stop using the medication. Within two weeks, the frequency of his headaches had declined by a startling 95 percent without the use of drugs. As Denny wrote, he "had a life again. It has now been five months and I remain 98 percent headache-free!"

The results were just as impressive for a patient named Walt. He had suffered from chronic pain for fifteen years, and despite taking many painkillers, he could not control his pain. Walt was referred to me by one of my colleagues, Gale Joslin, Ph.D., and I treated him with VT on the phone. His SUD declined from a 10 to a 4, and at that point, there were no remaining perturbations. But his SUD seemed stuck, unable to go lower. I suspected that we had a case of inertial delay.

Sure enough, four hours later, Walt called Dr. Joslin. He was absolutely exhilarated. His pain was gone, he exclaimed. He said he had not felt so good in nearly two decades!

Although the above examples of Walt and Denny involve physical ailments, the advanced generations of Thought Field Therapy are just as successful in the treatment of psychological disorders.

One of my colleagues treated a man in his sixties who had been in traditional psychotherapy for more than twenty years. He had been severely abused as a child and had carried the traumas from those early experiences with him his entire life. He was treated with Causal Diagnosis for just two hour-long sessions, and the emotional pain associated with those traumas was eliminated. As his TFT therapist said, "We accomplished in two sessions what twenty years of psychotherapy had been unable to achieve. Freud thought that no one over forty could even be helped, but we have certainly proven him wrong on that score."

In another case, a forty-seven-year-old woman named Beverly had lost her zest for life. Once vivacious, energetic, and a high achiever, she suddenly lost her motivation, and she described herself as being "stuck." Beverly canceled a vacation that she had been looking forward to, and her normally open communication with her husband ended. She felt that she had lost her purpose in life, and described herself as falling into an abyss. Her spirit, she said, was broken. (A problem such as this one, that appears to arise suddenly, has most likely been developing slowly—until it reaches a "critical mass." This buildup is sometimes due to the cumulative effect of toxins.)

Beverly was initially treated by a colleague of mine, who used the standard TFT algorithms for anxiety, depression, and trauma, among others—all without success. Then, after her therapist moved up to Causal Diagnosis, Beverly experienced at least brief periods of relief, lasting a few hours. Finally, I was asked to help Beverly by phone using Voice Technology.

I identified a toxin—coffee—and in less than twenty minutes, we were able to completely eliminate all of Beverly's remaining perturbations. At the same time, her "broken spirit" vanished. There was a glimmer in her eyes again. She told us that life was "incredibly worth living" once more. By the way, although she consumed less than one cup of coffee each morning, she agreed to go java-free in the future.

Most people will not need the advanced therapies. Remember, the success rate of the algorithms is 75 to 80 percent, so for most readers, this book will provide all the tools necessary to eliminate their psychological problems.

No therapy produces cures with the same regularity as Thought Field Therapy. Even if you haven't completely eradicated your problem after your first use of TFT, be persistent. Before long, you'll be able to get your own SUD score down to 1. In the process, you'll change your life forever.

7

THE APEX PROBLEM

EARLY IN THE development of Thought Field Therapy, I attended a meeting where a prominent author and acquaintance of mine—I'll call her Kelly—was scheduled to speak. Kelly's latest book had just been published, and she was eager to publicize it. At the same time, however, she dreaded public speaking. As she sat at the head table, waiting to be introduced to a ballroom filled with about 250 people, she fidgeted nervously in her chair.

At one point, Kelly rose to go to the ladies' room, and I stopped her in the hallway. She had lit up a cigarette and looked very frightened. "I'm just dying over this," she told me. Then she added, "I'd rather be boiled alive in oil than speak here today." She didn't seem to be exaggerating.

I told Kelly about the work I had been doing with Thought Field Therapy and that I might be able to help ease her anxiety, and do it quickly. At first, she didn't seem interested. But on her way back from the restroom, she gave in and agreed to let me work on easing her fear. She put out her cigarette, and as we stood in the hallway, I guided her through a TFT algorithm. She didn't appear particularly enthusiastic about the procedure and merely seemed to be putting up with it.

Within two minutes, however, after she returned to her table, I could see that a transformation had occurred. Kelly appeared completely free of the anxiety that had nearly debilitated her just moments earlier. She seemed confident and ready to take the lectern.

A few minutes later, standing on the podium, Kelly hit a home run. She was extremely relaxed. She spoke dynamically and with humor. From the beginning, the audience was captivated. She talked to them as though she were conversing with friends in her living room. Near the end of the lecture, she told the crowd that she was looking forward to giving more talks, and it appeared that she meant it. "This has been a wonderful experience," she said.

What a change! As Kelly returned to her seat, she received a lengthy and warm round of applause. Of course, I was absolutely delighted.

As the meeting adjourned, I approached Kelly to say good-bye and told her how much I enjoyed her lecture. Then I said, "I'm so glad that the treatment worked so well."

Kelly looked at me with a puzzled expression on her face. "What treatment? Roger, that wasn't a real treatment, was it? You didn't do anything."

Later, when Kelly's friends asked her how she had ever conquered her fear of public speaking, she said that it had simply gone away on its own. She didn't credit TFT with helping her in any way.

Kelly's reaction is not uncommon. In fact, it happens quite frequently with Thought Field Therapy. I call this phenomenon the Apex Problem.

WHAT'S THE APEX PROBLEM?

The Apex Problem occurs when a person's problem is eliminated, and he or she reports it is gone, but does not credit the treatment with producing the cure. I call it the Apex Problem because when it occurs, the mind is not functioning at its apex, or peak level. I borrowed the term from Arthur Koestler, the Hungarian-born British writer, who spoke of minds operating at their apex.

As I wrote in Chapter 3, TFT is counterintuitive. All of our lives, we've been taught that the only path to emotional healing is through weeks, months, or even years of emotionally painful psychotherapy. Even then, the chances of complete healing are remote at best. But TFT is different. In most cases, it requires just a single treatment that takes only minutes to perform. Once an individual's perturbations are collapsed, the psychological problem that may have been present for years will disappear, typically for good.

When people are treated successfully with TFT, they're often like Kelly—they recognize that their emotional turmoil is gone but can't believe such a simple technique could possibly be responsible for their rapid and complete healing. They'll acknowledge that they've never felt better, but they do not credit the treatment for this improvement. TFT just seems implausible. How, they ask, could tapping on points along energy meridians cure something in minutes that has caused so much anguish for so many years?

"Was I Really in Pain?"

The healing with TFT is so dramatic and so complete that clients sometimes actually deny that they ever had any anger or anxiety or other emotional distress in the first place. Even though they sought help for their psychological turmoil and gave it a high rating on the SUD scale when the treatment began, they suddenly wonder whether they ever really had a problem. They might say something like, "I feel so good now that I must not have been depressed after all."

I often suggest that patients tape-record their TFT session. Later, if they have any doubts that they really had an emotional problem, or about how they ranked its severity on the SUD scale, they'll have the tape to confirm that it really existed and was eliminated in a single, brief therapy session. The tape recording, if they listen to it, makes it more difficult for them to spontaneously "rewrite history," and to forget that they had once been in emotional pain.

Other clients have told me that they viewed the aftermath of TFT differently. They believed that their emotional problem still existed, but that TFT had somehow suppressed it. One woman, after rating her post-treatment SUD at 1, explained it away by saying, "Well, it's still an underlying thing; it's just not on the surface anymore." (Before the TFT treatment, however, she had never described it that way.)

Some people have said that they haven't credited Thought Field Therapy for their healing because to do so, they'd have to consider TFT something of a "miracle." As they understand psychological problems and their treatment, TFT is difficult for them to accept. The first time you saw or experienced TFT, it may have seemed rather miraculous. (In this instance, *miracle* is defined as something that happens contrary to our expectations or what we believe we ought to expect. Writer-scientist Arthur C. Clarke, co-author of Stanley Kubrick's *2001: A Space Odyssey*, described his third law this way: "Any sufficiently advanced technology is indistinguishable from magic."

The Apex Problem is a way in which individuals can avoid carefully evaluating what has taken place, which would require rethinking old beliefs about psychological distress and its proper treatment.

The most common Apex Problem is when treated people say: "You distracted me, and now I cannot think of my problem." It is impossible to say those words, however, and *not* think of the problem. My first response to a statement such as this one is: "Well, you are not being distracted now, so let's see if you can get upset." The typical reply is, "No, I'm unable to get upset now. So I must not be able to think about it."

Each time people like this thought about their problems in the past, they would become terribly upset, often soaring to a 10 on the SUD scale. But after being treated successfully with TFT, they find themselves unable to get upset, and therefore wrongly conclude that they must not be thinking of the problem. Because this form of the Apex Problem happens so frequently, I put a sign in my office that states, in very large type, "I CAN'T THINK ABOUT THE PROBLEM!" In fact, a more accurate statement was written directly underneath the original one: "What I mean is that now, after the treatment, I am unable to become upset when I think about it."

What the Research Shows

There is some interesting research related to the Apex Problem. Studies have compared the functions of the two hemispheres of the brain, and one investigator, Michael S. Gazzaniga of Dartmouth College, has described what he calls the "left-brain interpreter." He has found that the left brain will create "explanations" for phenomena unfamiliar to it, even though there is *absolutely no factual basis* for that explanation. In fact, the explanation is irrelevant, completely removed from what really has happened.

This may be what's happening in response to TFT. The left brain is being presented with something it cannot understand (the rapid, successful treatment of an emotional problem), and so it creates explanations of its own that are contrary to what has really taken place. These rationalizations become so powerful that they override all critical thinking. Some psychologists call this *cognitive dissonance*.

Several years ago, I appeared on a television talk show with the chairman of the department of psychiatry at a major university who was a recognized expert on phobias. Although he made some complimentary remarks about my book *The Five Minute Phobia Cure*, he believed that my therapeutic approach could never truly help people with phobias because, as he said, fears are almost never cured with *any* kind of treatment.

I was unfazed by the comments. On live television and in front of the doctor, I began to treat three volunteers whom he had characterized as "severe phobics." One of them was a woman so terrified of heights that she lived in a basement. After TFT, however, she climbed a ladder that had been placed on the stage. At that point, she described herself as phobia-free. Then I treated another woman who was afraid of spiders. Within minutes, she held a tarantula in her palm in full view of the TV cameras. The third patient, who claimed that she often fainted at the mere thought of cats, held a furry feline in her lap following TFT, while her husband, who was in the studio audience, looked on with amazement.

Rather than acknowledge the power of what he had just witnessed, the psychiatry professor ran for cover. He retreated to a position that TFT's "cures" were produced by "showbiz." (Mind you, he had not asserted beforehand that phobics could be cured by "showbiz," whatever that is.) He refused to acknowledge that TFT had resolved these phobias.

DO YOU NEED TO BELIEVE?

Until now, most psychologists believed that their treatments required the confidence or optimism of their patients in order to work. If a patient didn't believe in the treatment, it wasn't going to be effective. But with Thought Field Therapy, this isn't the case at all. If you're skeptical about whether TFT can really produce psychological or physical improvement, it won't interfere with the power of this approach.

One of the most interesting examples of the Apex Problem occurred with a surgeon named James. He was in his mid-fifties, and thirty years earlier, when he was a medical student, he had been diagnosed with melanoma. The malignant skin lesion was removed, but despite the successful treatment, James began constantly checking for signs of another skin cancer in order to excise it immediately. It became a disturbing compulsion. Even the slightest blemish created so much anxiety that he could barely function until he surgically removed the blemish.

Before long, James recognized that he had an emotional problem. He got into psychoanalysis and over the years spent a phenomenal $300,000 trying to resolve it. But the therapy didn't work. "I learned a lot about myself," James told me, "but all that self-examination did nothing to get rid of the compulsion. It was still there after all those years in therapy and all that cost."

Then James was introduced to Thought Field Therapy. He received three brief TFT treatments directed toward eliminating this compulsion. They seemed to work. But James was skeptical. "It's too simplistic," he said. "It's so strange."

That was the last I heard from James for three years. Then I received an unexpected phone call from him. "I haven't had any trace of the compulsion since the treatment," James said. "I haven't been preoccupied with melanoma at all." Then, almost apologetically, he told me that it had taken him all this time to put the entire picture together. He finally realized not only that his compulsion was gone, but that the Apex Problem had kept him from recognizing how TFT had eliminated the problem.

Some therapists now ask their patients to prepare for this kind of reaction to TFT. They advise their clients to expect to be surprised and even shocked by experiencing a complete, rapid recovery. By anticipating this disbelief and denial, they will be much more understanding of the dramatic changes that TFT can produce.

IS IT A MATTER OF DISTRACTION?

It's not hard to be impressed by Thought Field Therapy. After all, when you've been unable to quit smoking for decades, or when you've had a fear of dogs all your life, you should find it really quite remarkable to conquer the problem in minutes with TFT. But for the reasons I've already discussed, some people seek an explanation other than Thought Field Therapy that might be more in sync with their own belief system. After being successfully treated, quite a few individuals respond by saying, "I think you distracted me!"

Here's what they've told me: They feel that the mere act of proceeding through the algorithm, in which tapping and other maneuvers are the focus of the treatment, has taken their mind off their emotional turmoil. In due time, they say, it will all come rushing back. This is another Apex Problem response.

Of course, they're wrong. Distraction is the *furthest* thing from what really happens. TFT, in fact, does just the opposite. With the algorithms, you are instructed to "tune," or think about, the particular problem you are trying to treat, not distract yourself from it!

I recall a recent case in which one of my TFT trainees was working with a depressed client and had asked me to supervise the treatment over the phone. Using the advanced TFT technique called Voice Technology, I identified the optimal treatments for the patient, and my trainee administered them.

The client, whom I'll call Theresa, had been a 9 on the SUD scale when the treatment began. Afterward, she said there had been no improvement, which puzzled me. I conducted additional voice analysis, which showed no evidence of any remaining perturbations. So we asked Theresa again whether she was sure that she still felt depressed. She thought about it for a moment and then responded, "Well, I don't feel depressed right now. But I think I've been distracted for a few minutes, and I'm sure I'll feel depressed tomorrow. So I decided not to report any change."

I reminded Theresa that we wanted to know how she was feeling *at that moment*, which she finally admitted was a 1 on the SUD scale. In all likelihood, that was how she would continue to feel from that time forward.

Distraction is actually an accepted technique in behavioral therapy, but it is thoroughly ineffective. Most psychotherapists understand this. Even so, feeling they have nowhere else to turn, some still fall back on the distraction explanation for TFT, as do their clients.

If the "distraction" argument doesn't ring true, many people will try something else—*anything* else! I recall working with a client named Lois who was overwhelmed by phobias—particularly, a fear of driving. Although she had wanted to get behind the wheel of a car for about ten years, each time she thought of doing so, she would go to pieces. Just *thinking* about driving propelled her SUD score to a 10.

I treated Lois with Thought Field Therapy. When we were done, I asked her to turn her attention back to driving and determine her new SUD score. Suddenly, she said, "Oh, I can't do that right now."

"Well, just take a few moments to think about driving. See if you become as upset now as you did before the treatment."

Lois paused for a few moments and seemed to be trying to follow my instructions. Then she said, "Well, I'm not getting upset right now. But that's because you distracted me with all that tapping."

I reminded Lois that she was no longer tapping or performing the other components of the algorithm. Even if she were being distracted during the treatment itself (which she wasn't), it was now over. She should be able to get a sense of whether there was any lingering fear associated with thoughts of driving.

Lois said she'd try again to get in touch with any anxiety that remained. After about twenty to thirty seconds of silence, she finally said there wasn't any left. However, she seemed uncomfortable with her response, and she quickly interjected, "But, of course, I'm not upset *now* because I'm just sitting here talking to you. If I were driving, it might be different."

I reminded Lois that just a few minutes earlier, before the TFT treatment, she had rated her fear at a 10 on the SUD scale. Just *thinking* about driving had caused her anxiety to soar.

What was happening with Lois? Like other clients, she simply couldn't accept the fact that a therapy as unusual as TFT could eliminate problems that had bothered her for a decade—even though TFT was formulated with the express purpose of eradicating just that kind of distress.

IS IT JUST THE PLACEBO EFFECT?

You've probably heard of the placebo effect. Briefly, it's a phenomenon in which healing is purported to occur not because the treatment being offered is powerful, but because the patient and/or doctor *believe* that it is. A person may be given nothing more than a sugar pill, but if he thinks that the pill is or might be a potent drug instead, his condition may improve. Even so, although it is presumed that the placebo effect is the cause of some cures, placebo-induced cure rates have been found to be dubious.

How does Thought Field Therapy fit into this scenario? Some clients, and more predictably many skeptical psychotherapists, have told me that TFT's improvements are simply the placebo effect at work. These same therapists, however, have conceded that they've never seen a trauma or an equally serious problem eliminated by the placebo effect. In fact, recent reports have raised doubts about the validity of the placebo effect altogether. This is another form of the Apex Problem, if a more rational one. Clearly, TFT is much more than the placebo effect. Consider the fact that in its most advanced forms, TFT is successful 97 to 99 percent of the time—a much higher rate than even extravagant claims of a placebo effect.

When I treated Mary, my very first TFT patient, I was so amazed by the results that at the time I thought perhaps it was the placebo effect at work. But conditions then were no more conducive to a placebo effect than they are today. I didn't believe in the treatment back then—I didn't even know it was a treatment. Mary didn't believe in the treatment either, nor did she know it was a treatment. But even though we had neither a believing doctor nor a believing patient, the therapy worked, just as it has for many thousands of people since.

Because of the skepticism with which some clients and psychologists view Thought Field Therapy, I've often said that we don't get our fair share of so-called placebo cures (not that we really need them!). We are constantly working against negative expectations rather than being the beneficiaries of positive ones. Even if the placebo effect exists, a precondition for placebo success is a deep belief in the therapeutic technique by the client and/or the doctor (preferably both). But many people approach TFT with a militant disbelief that the technique could ever be effective. Despite the intensity of this skepticism, TFT still works.

WHY THE APEX PROBLEM IS IMPORTANT

Some naive therapists have told me that they don't see the Apex Problem as a problem at all. One colleague, a therapist named Charles, has described what he calls "the benevolent Apex Problem" (where *benevolent* means "harmless"). He told me about a client with chronic, severe back pain. She had already been to many pain clinics, been evaluated by a dozen pain specialists, and taken every kind of painkiller in the doctors' black bag. Finally, she was contemplating undergoing high-risk spinal surgery that, if complications occurred, might leave her paralyzed. Charles treated her with TFT—and to the woman's surprise, her pain was completely eliminated. How did she respond? Of course, she was delighted. Then she told Charles, "I think those medications have finally started working!" Charles was surprised by her reaction but didn't try to change her mind. He simply thought of it as a benevolent Apex Problem.

I disagree, however. If the pain should return, this woman is likely to have that risky surgery or continue taking ineffective and expensive medications rather than return for a TFT "tune-up." There's really nothing benevolent about that. She needs to understand what treatment helped her so if the problem recurs, she'll know where to seek effective help again.

Thus, while the Apex Problem *won't* interfere with the success of your treatment with TFT, it may influence how you react to it. Quite remarkably, the most advanced forms of TFT have a higher success rate than penicillin, even in the drug's heyday before resistant strains weakened its power significantly. If TFT has reduced or eliminated your problem, but you find that you're not celebrating, the Apex Problem is the explanation. You may need to do some mental work at the apex of your mind to completely understand and acknowledge the reality and the power of TFT.

On occasion, I have clients who actually become hostile once their emotional distress has been successfully treated by TFT. They react as though I have played some kind of practical joke on them. It reminds me of something that a skilled magician once told me. He said that at times, when he performed an unbelievable magic trick, someone in the audience would react antagonistically. He asked for my professional opinion on what was happening there, and I told him that perhaps people like this had inferiority feelings. Believing that they *ought* to know how the trick had been done, they may have felt inadequate or even stupid that they didn't. This could be one explanation for the Apex Problem—people just can't understand how a treatment like TFT could be successful and feel foolish because of it.

Here's the bottom line: with or without the Apex Problem, the results produced by TFT are exciting and fulfilling. If you've been in traditional psychotherapy, you know how frustrating that experience can be. With TFT, however, even when the Apex Problem is at play, you'll experience results much more powerful and more rapid than with any other kind of treatment.

8

SOME CLOSING THOUGHTS

In August 1998, one of my professional colleagues, Jenny Edwards, was conducting a two-week TFT training program in Kenya. In the midst of one of those sessions, she received word of a devastating terrorist bombing at the U.S. embassy in downtown Nairobi, about twenty minutes from the training site. A stunning 257 people were killed by the massive blast, and more than 5,000 people were injured.

Jenny joined some of her trainees at Kenyatta Hospital to tend to the bombing victims. She wondered whether Thought Field Therapy could possibly work for patients who had experienced such severe emotional trauma, not to mention such serious physical wounds. She also had some other basic concerns, including whether it would be appropriate to ask people whose faces were filled with stitches and bandages to tap on their eyebrows and under their eyes to self-administer TFT (in cases like these, we can actually use alternate points on the toes).

As Jenny moved through the hospital, she stopped at the bedside of a woman in horrific pain—a 10 on a 0-to-10 SUD scale (some of our trainees use an 11-point scale)—from lower body injuries. Even the most potent pain medications had no effect on her discomfort. After a few minutes of building rapport with the woman, Jenny told her, "I have something that *might* help you. I'm not sure it will work. It would involve tapping on particular places on your body and would take about five minutes. I'm willing to try if you would like me to."

The patient reacted quickly. "I'll do anything. I'm in so much pain." Then she added, "I also keep thinking a bomb will explode any minute in the hospital. I know it's probably not going to happen; however, I can't get the thought out of my mind!"

Jenny began administering the pain algorithm. As they moved through it together, the patient's pain level dropped significantly, with her SUD declining from a 10 to a 5. However, it wouldn't move lower, even after treatment for a psychological reversal. So Jenny shifted to the trauma algorithm. After the series of tapping and other maneuvers, the patient's SUD for trauma had declined rapidly from 10 to 0. Next, Jenny repeated the pain algorithm. This time, with the trauma completely resolved, the woman's SUD for pain dipped to 0 as well. In minutes, the physical pain and the emotional trauma were completely gone.

As the afternoon unfolded, Jenny helped other patients as well. One woman, whose trauma and pain were both 10 on the SUD scale, was staring into space when Jenny approached her. She had a heavily bandaged arm; her hand was limp. Then the trauma algorithm was administered. Almost immediately, the patient's SUD for trauma plummeted all the way to 0, with no psychological reversal. Then Jenny turned her attention to the woman's physical pain. As the patient tapped according to Jenny's instructions, her discomfort fell to a 0, too. Color returned to her face. She was able to move her hand again. Amazingly, she even smiled and laughed for the first time since the bombing.

TFT: A THERAPY FOR THE NEW MILLENNIUM

These dramatic examples show what is possible with Thought Field Therapy. TFT has been called the "power therapy" of the new century. With a track record now spanning two decades, this remarkable therapy has cured many thousands of people of their psychological (and in some cases, physical) problems in just minutes.

Early in this book, I promised that you could make dramatic changes in your overall psychological health by using the brief but effective TFT algorithms. If you've followed the simple instructions in these pages, you have probably already experienced rapid healing in your life. Even if you were skeptical early on, you've seen how TFT can relieve problems that may have lingered for years, from phobias to addictive urges, from anger to guilt, from shame to depression. As you've worked with these techniques, you've seen that they don't require unique skills to implement—everything most people need has been presented right here. The algorithms are simple to learn and easy to use.

You've probably had to change your mindset about psychological disorders and their treatment. No longer are you required to make numerous visits to a therapist's office, reliving the painful events in your past to move toward healing. The solutions are within your reach within minutes. With TFT, you can identify the disturbed Thought Field and remove the causal elements of the disturbance. In the process, you will experience the collapse of that disturbance. Psychological upsets are eliminated quickly, simply by tapping on carefully chosen treatment points that can rebalance the body's energy system and stimulate a genuine transformation in your well-being.

For many years I practiced traditional psychotherapy. Too often, I still see it do more harm than good. In the TFT era, I treated a middle-aged man named Phillip who had a severe fear of bridges. He had been treated five years earlier by a behavioral psychologist who had coerced him to drive over a lengthy bridge. When Phillip's car reached the other side of the long span, the therapist declared him cured! After all, he had successfully maneuvered his car from one end of the bridge to the other. For his psychotherapist, that was all that was necessary to consider the treatment a success. He never even bothered to ask Phillip how he felt!

But I did ask Phillip that question when he called me for help. His answer: "I felt absolutely terrible." In fact, he was so traumatized by the experience of driving across the bridge that he had refused to try any additional therapy since. When he finally did seek my help, I knew it was absolutely crucial to monitor his distress level—and as we began, he told me it was a 10 on the SUD scale. In the ensuing minutes, we dealt not only with his fear of bridges, but also the trauma. Predictably, TFT worked immediately. We eliminated the perturbations and his SUD rating showed that there was absolutely no distress remaining. Best of all, Phillip said he felt "just great."

THE NEXT GENERATION OF TFT

The success that you enjoy with the self-help elements of Thought Field Therapy should be permanent. But if you notice a problem returning, consider contacting a TFT practitioner. He or she can help you determine whether a toxin is responsible for the resurrection of your problem and help you identify that toxin and eliminate it from your life.

Keep in mind that advanced TFT therapies are also available (see Chapter 6). Voice Technology, the most sophisticated level of Thought Field Therapy, has successfully resolved the most difficult cases, time after time, and it can do the same for you. Voice Technology is achieving the highest success rates in psychotherapy today. For example:

• Not long ago, I helped one of my trainees manage a patient who had suffered from depression for thirteen years and had taken antidepressants for most of that time. My colleague had been able to reduce the client's depression from a 10 to a 5 on the SUD scale, but could not get it lower. I advised using Voice Technology, which proved to be very useful. Within minutes, Voice Technology had revealed and collapsed multiple perturbations. The client said his SUD rating had plummeted to a 1, indicating that his problem had been eliminated. For the first time in more than a decade, he felt completely free of depression.

• Sam was a concentration camp survivor who had lived with the trauma of that horrible experience for more than fifty years. He had lost his entire family in Auschwitz, and, understandably, his mental health had been shattered. His inner turmoil defined him not only during his waking hours, but even while he slept. He described having had nightmares every night for decades. "Even though I was physically freed from Auschwitz as a young man," he said, "I'm still an emotional prisoner of the camp."

Sam had seen me speaking about TFT on a television talk show and made an appointment. I administered a three-minute treatment and waited for him to react. Almost immediately, he said he felt better. More important, when I spoke with him in the weeks and months that followed, the misery that had overwhelmed his life for so long was gone. For the first time, he could talk about his concentration camp experience without becoming upset. The nightmares were gone as well. As generally happens with traumas from many years ago, Sam enjoyed permanent healing with TFT. (The ease of my treatment should not minimize the horrors and evil of concentration camps, rapes, or muggings; these crimes still clearly demonstrate the horrors that humans can inflict on others.)

• At a behavioral medicine conference, I treated an eighty-two-year-old woman named Miriam with TFT before an audience of health-care professionals. She had spent several years caring for her husband, who had been ill with Alzheimer's disease. In addition to the physical and emotional demands of providing his day-to-day care, Miriam supported him during his very slow and agonizing death. She couldn't get those painful images out of her mind. Not only did they constantly haunt her, but she also developed a physical shaking disorder in reaction to the psychological stress in her life.

Miriam had come to the conference in hopes of finding something that might relieve her chronic suffering. I treated her with a brief TFT session in front of the large group of therapists. In minutes, her perturbations were eliminated. She also stopped shaking. The audience was stunned at the ease with which her severe agony had been eliminated.

A CUTTING-EDGE TREATMENT

I believe that Thought Field Therapy is on the cutting edge of a new era in healing, and not just for psychological problems. As I've described in this book, exciting research with Heart Rate Variability (HRV) technology has measured the dramatic *physiological* changes that TFT can produce in the autonomic nervous system. HRV has shown that as psychological healing is taking place with TFT, physiological improvements are occurring as well. This has enormous implications for reducing stress levels, producing internal homeostasis, and stimulating healing in many areas, from heart arrhythmias to chronic illnesses. Remember, nothing seems capable of improving HRV readings as rapidly and effectively as Thought Field Therapy—an extremely important finding, since HRV is a powerful indicator of an individual's overall health.

During the last twenty years, I've had the privilege of personally training hundreds of new TFT practitioners and treating many thousands of their clients with difficult problems using the techniques described in this book. More people are learning about and using Thought Field Therapy than ever before. In fact, tens of thousands of people worldwide have discovered that there is no need to suffer with an emotional disturbance any longer, whether it has bothered them for just a few weeks or for most of their life. TFT provides the tools for permanent healing.

Although you may have found some of the concepts of TFT—from Thought Fields to perturbations—hard to grasp at first, I trust that any misgivings have vanished as you've noticed dramatic and positive changes in your own well-being. It is reassuring to know that you now have the ability to tap the healer within and experience emotional (and perhaps physical) renewal, quickly and safely. TFT can provide predictable healing and, in turn, significant improvements in your life.

Each of us has the power to build the life we want. Thanks to the personal journey that led to Thought Field Therapy, I have been intellectually stimulated and scientifically rewarded. Along the way, TFT has helped many people live happier, healthier, and more meaningful lives.

The power of TFT is right in your own hands—quite literally—and with it the power to transform your own personal journey and to achieve the life you want. I wish you good luck and good health.

APPENDIX

HOW TO FIND PROFESSIONALS WHO HAVE APPROVED TRAINING IN CALLAHAN TECHNIQUES THOUGHT FIELD THERAPY

THERE ARE A growing number of people who falsely claim to be trained in Callahan Techniques Thought Field Therapy (CTTFT), so it is important to check with our organization in order to find professionals who are adequately and properly trained in our procedures. There are now professionals with approved training not only throughout the United States but also in Canada, the UK, Australia, France, Mexico, Italy, Germany, South America, and Japan. For general information and to find an approved CTTFT therapist in your location, please call our office in California at 760-360-7832.

Visit our website to find professionals who are trained at our highest level (Voice Technology). Those trained at this level are able to help people over the phone wherever the patient is located. Our website can be found at www.tftrx.com.

We now have a very exciting home study course which teaches not only our algorithms but also the principles of Causal Diagnosis. Call our office or contact our website for more information.

CONTACT INFORMATION

For the last half century, Dr. Callahan has researched and developed simple and effective self-help procedures to assist you with the challenges and stresses of daily life. Based on this continual research and development, he has created many simple algorithms for your use. Most of Dr. Callahan's products are not available in stores, so for more information about these products or the revolutionary new findings in Heart Rate Variability, call, write, fax, or visit our websites:

Dr. Roger J. Callahan
Callahan Techniques, Ltd.
Thought Field Therapy Training Center
78-816 Via Carmel
La Quinta, CA 92253
Phone: 800-359-CURE (2873)
Fax: 760-360-5258
Phone for international inquiries: 001-760-564-1008
www.selfhelpuniv.com (self-help site)
www.tftrx.com (professional site)

For information on home training in Callahan Techniques Thought Field Therapy:

Step A—Basic TFT Training Self-Study Course
Presented by Dr. Roger J. Callahan, founder of TFT, this course teaches the step-by-step process for determining precise protocols for whatever the presenting problems are and uses the same methods by which all of the algorithms were developed. It includes the training manual, two training videos, one demonstrational video, six audiotapes, and our new Handheld Flip Chart, and it costs $499. For more information about Step A or any of our other training programs, contact us at the numbers given above.

Newsletter—The Thought Field
Subscriptions cost $27 for four issues in the United States and $29 for foreign subscriptions.

INDEX

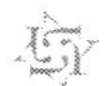